HOW TO WRITE
MEANINGFUL
STANDARDS OF CARE

HOW TO WRITE MEANINGFUL STANDARDS OF CARE

THIRD EDITION

Elizabeth J. Mason, Ph.D., R.N.
International Consultant
Nursing Standards
Quality Improvement

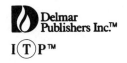

Delmar Publishers Inc.™

I(T)P™

NOTICE TO THE READER

Cover design by Michael Traylor

Delmar Staff
  Publisher: David Gordon
  Associate Editor: Elisabeth F. Williams
  Project Manager: Carol Micheli
  Production Coordinator: Jennifer Gaines
  Design Coordinator: Michael Traylor
  Production Services: Susan Geraghty

For information, address Delmar Publishers Inc., 3 Columbia Circle, Box 15015, Albany, NY 12212

Library of Congress Cataloging-in-Publication Data

Mason, Elizabeth J.
    How to write meaningful standards of care / Elizabeth J. Mason.
       p. cm.
    Rev. ed. of: How to write meaningful nursing standards. 2nd ed.
  ©1984.
    Includes bibliographical references and index.
    ISBN 0-8273-5316-2 (pb)
    1. Nursing—Standards. 2. Nursing—Authorship. I. Mason,
  Elizabeth J. How to write meaningful nursing standards. II. Title.
    [DNLM: 1. Nursing Care—standards—outlines. 2. Writing—
    outlines. WY 18 M398h 1994]
  RT85.5.M37   1994
  808'.06661—dc20
  DNLM/DLC
  for Library of Congress   93–5210
                                                                         CIP

Contents

Preface
to the
Third Edition

Every job is a self-portrait of
the person who did it.
Autograph your work with
excellence!
—Author unknown

I believe this poem is germane to the era of quality management and quality improvement, an era I have been working toward since 1972. While I am excited that this era has arrived, health professionals and administrators in health care organizations still need to change many of the ideas and values they have held for their entire career. Even though there is a great struggle ahead, I believe the results are worth the effort. The results are that patients will experience positive outcomes more consistently, and those who work in health care organizations will experience a lowering of the "hassle level,"[1] both welcome changes. As in the first two editions, this book is written to assist health professionals, including nurses, to write standards of care.

During the last 10 years since the second edition was published there has been an explosion of changes in the delivery of health care. Despite the changes the structure of the method I've developed for writing standards is unchanged. This method can assist any clinician in any health care setting to write standards of care. In tests conducted by the author, clinicians can write the process, content and outcome standards for a procedure or unit of care in 30 minutes or less. The changes in the book relate to the new concepts in application of the method and recommendations for implementing the standards. Topics that have been added since the last edition include:

1. How to write standards for Interdisciplinary Units of Care
2. A method for establishing the efficiency of the standards
3. Recommendations for implementing the standards
4. Examples of standards for use in various settings

I have made some semantic changes in the text. In the second edition the term *client* appeared to be emerging in the literature over the term *patient*. Although there are many terms to refer to a consumer of health care, the literature at present is favoring *patient*; thus, *patient* is being used to refer to all the terms relating to consumers of health care. This is true also of *family* and *significant others*. You will see the word *family* throughout the book to mean both significant others, as well as family. There are authors who define the type of standards in this book as standards of practice or standards of care. Because *standards of care* is used more frequently to relate to the care of patients (*standards of practice* definitions frequently include standards for a specific profession in addition to those standards that relate to the care of patients), I have used *standards of care* throughout the book. Lastly, in chapter 8, because the definitions in the literature were very similar for the terms *quality management* and *quality improvement*, I have used the terms interchangeably.

As in previous editions, this book is designed as a workbook providing a step-by-step approach to writing standards. Specific examples of standards are provided, highlighting the features that make the quality of care measurable.

Elizabeth J. Mason

NOTE

1. Crosby, P.B. *Quality without tears*, p. 154. New York: McGraw-Hill, 1984.

Preface
to the
Second Edition

The major goal that guided the writing of the first edition of this book is the same for the second: to assist nurses in writing valid, meaningful standards for nursing care. During the six years since the publication of the first edition, many changes in the requirements of accrediting agencies and third-party payers have affected the quality of nursing care. The Joint Commission on the Accreditation of Hospitals has made the requirements for accreditation more extensive and specific; and with the passage of the Tax Equity and Fiscal Responsibility Act of 1982 and the reimbursement in some states for hospitalization by diagnostic related groups (DRGs), payment for nursing care is based on the client's medical diagnosis. As a result, there is today an even greater need for nurses in health care agencies to develop standards to guarantee the quality of nursing care.

Because of changes in reimbursement for health care, there is also a great need to identify the true cost of providing quality nursing care. Many methods are currently being proposed to estimate the cost of nursing care, but the true cost of quality nursing care can be identified only when standards of nursing care are used to plan nursing care and develop staffing patterns. When standards of nursing care are developed, the level of nursing personnel required to implement the standards can be specified, and if the standards are written in the proper format, a computer can be used to compile individualized care plans for clients and to determine the cost of the nursing care administered.

The second edition of *How to Write Meaningful Nursing Standards* incorporates helpful suggestions from the many users and reviewers of the first edition. The method of writing standards has not been altered, but some of the steps are described in greater detail, and the organizational format has been streamlined. The major change in this edition is the introduction of the *unit of nursing care:* the cluster of process, outcome, and content standards that define the nursing care for a given nursing diagnosis, health problem, or need; a definable point on the health-illness-health continuum; or a specific developmental stage. The unit of nursing care is vital to developing individualized nursing care plans for clients, evaluating the specific nursing care administered to clients, staffing a nursing unit, and establishing the true cost of nursing care.

Chapter 1 has been reorganized and expanded to meet the needs of nurses responsible for organizing others to write standards. Some of the definitions of concepts have been clarified and new concepts have been introduced. The uses of standards are described in relation to the various steps in the nursing process, staffing, job descriptions, and the policies of the health care agency. In Chapters 2 and 3, the sections on writing of standards for a nursing intervention have been simplified and clarified, and two practice examples have been included. The last portions of Chapters 2 and 3 have been refocused on developing standards for a unit of nursing care rather than for a nursing care plan. Nurses can use units of nursing care to individualize care, as opposed to developing "canned" care plans that are not flexible in meeting the changing needs of clients. Chapter 6 has been expanded and revised, particularly the sections on resource persons, implementing a plan for developing standards, and packaging standards. The section on resources has been amplified to include the types of administrative support nurses need to complete the task of writing standards, especially for a large division or agency.

It is my hope that the second edition retains the strengths of the first while incorporating relevant information to meet the challenges of providing quality nursing care in an environment of diminishing resources.

Elizabeth J. Mason

Preface
to the
First Edition

Standards are essential to the nursing profession because they define un-
equivocally what *quality* nursing care is and provide specific criteria that can
be used to determine whether quality care has been provided. Too often
nurses implement standards that are implied. In this era of accountability,
nurses must formulate standards that are concrete and understandable to
other nurses, health care professionals, accrediting agencies, and consumers.

The standards developed by the American Nurses' Association are not
explicit enough to be implemented; hence, the quality of care defined by
these "standards" cannot be evaluated. The same is true of most books and
monographs that list standards.

Even though standards have been written for several years, until now a
method has not been devised to develop standards that meet the following
criteria:

1. The standard is *explicit* and therefore meaningful to the nurse who
   must actually implement it.
2. The *quality* of nursing care defined by the standard can be evaluated

This book was written to ease the frustrations of nurses whose responsibility it is to write nursing standards that prescribe quality of care, and to
write them in such a way that the quality can be evaluated. By following the
step-by-step method described herein, these nurses can not only write new

standards but also rewrite ambiguous standards so as to make them particular and clear to those who must implement them. This method should also be assistive to both undergraduate and graduate nursing students.

This text is designed as a workbook, providing a step-by-step approach to writing substantial process standards, outcome standards, and content standards for nursing care. Specific examples of actual standards are provided, highlighting the features that make the quality of care defined by them measurable. Also, for those nurses who need to design a plan for writing nursing standards for a unit, a division, or an entire health care agency, a chapter devoted especially to this task is included.

Elizabeth J. Mason

Acknowledgments

In the previous editions the contributors were nurses in acute care facilities in the United States. In this edition I want to acknowledge the contributions of nurses in Australia and Great Britain as well as nurses in the United States who are working in various clinical settings. In addition, I have been working with health professionals other than nurses; their contributions provide an interdisciplinary flavor to this edition. All these committed health professionals are working diligently to ensure patients experience positive outcomes.

I also want to acknowledge the pioneers in the fields of Interdisciplinary Planning and Quality Management/Quality Improvement whose ideas I embrace. They have contributed ideas and strategies to assist management to provide the structure and support essential for clinicians to do their work.

I want to acknowledge Catherine Rosensteel for her creative writing and editing skills that enriched the text . . . and for her patience and kindness during the long editing sessions and the times I was struggling to explain a new idea.

Writing is a solitary and sometimes difficult activity for me. In order to immerse myself in the content, my family members greatly contributed to my well-being. For my aunt, Elizabeth Luman, I want to express my gratitude and admiration for the way she managed our home and tolerated the long periods of my silence while the computer hummed. My thanks to Barry Rosensteel who is quietly supportive and provides the know-how when mechanical items in my world malfunction. To my nephew, Shawn Rosen-steel, I am grateful he is such an important part of my life; his outlook on and approach to the world constantly enlighten and delight me. Thank you to John and Jean Luman for their welcome encouragement. And, I thank Gigi, my insistent-for-attention cockapoo, for providing chuckles daily.

This book is dedicated to Dr. William and Mrs. Margaret Luman Mason—their contributions to healthcare were truly a portrait in excellence!

1
What Is a Standard?

Quality health care is the implementation of the interventions and observations with associated goals provided to patients that meet their needs and result in positive outcomes for them. Health professionals require a system for assessing, planning, implementing, and evaluating health care that guarantees positive outcomes for every patient. Three vital components of such a system are the **process**, **content**, and **outcome standards** that define the quality of care.

DEFINITIONS

A **standard** is a valid definition of the quality of health care. To guarantee quality, every standard must be valid—that is, health care administered according to a standard will result in positive outcome(s) for patients. A standard is not valid unless it is precise; that is, all staff implementing and evaluating care understand the meaning of the standard.

Omitting the specificity from a standard would be like eliminating the inch indicators from a yardstick. Each person using the yardstick would have to estimate the length of an inch or foot, and thus, the accuracy of the measurement would vary greatly. Valid standards, on the other hand, are precise. Their meaning is shared by those who implement them as well as those who write them. Only valid, explicit standards can be used to evaluate the quality of health care.

Standards must be written so that they can be applied to the care provided in a specific clinical setting and with a specific health team. For example, the principles in the standards for a specific procedure used in an acute care or home care setting can be the same, but the setting and the equipment, as well as the level of practitioner who might be implementing the procedure, can affect the specific definition of the standards. This will be illustrated throughout the book.

Standards can be written in two formats: a unit of care or a procedure. A **unit of care** is the cluster of process (interventions/observations), content, and outcome standards that define the care related to:

- A specific nursing diagnosis, health problem, or patient care need
- A definable point on the health-illness-health continuum
- A specific stage of development

Some units of care are designed and implemented by a single health discipline. The method for writing standards for this type of unit of care is found in chapters 2 and 3. Other units of care contain the interventions and observations from more than one health discipline; these are interdisciplinary units of care. The method for writing these units of care is found in chapter 4.

A **procedure** contains the process standards and outcome standards that define what must be done to:

- Alter the patient's internal or external environment for the patient's benefit
- Assist the patient in coping with or changing the patient's environment
- Teach the patient how to cope with or prevent a health problem
- Involve the patient's family in assisting the patient in coping with or preventing a health problem
- Increase the psychological or physiological comfort of the patient
- Coordinate the provision of the health care needed by the patient with other members of the health team

There are three types of standards in a unit of care required to define the quality of health care: **process, outcome,** and **content.**

Process Standards

Process standards[1] define the quality of health care that is implemented. Process standards are the interventions, observations, and principles that must be done to guarantee positive outcomes for patients. Process standards should be developed for all procedures and units of care. Chapter 2 describes the process for writing process standards.

Content Standards

Content standards[2] define the substance of health care that is communicated to others and the substance of nurses' decisions. Content standards should be written for:

- Assessment
- Teaching
- Therapeutic communication
- Decision-making in emergency situations
- Documentation
- Reporting

Chapter 5 describes the method for writing content standards.

Outcome Standards

Outcome standards[3] define the expected change in the patient's health status and environment after receiving care and the extent of the patient's satisfaction with health care. Both positive and negative outcomes can result from health care. Positive outcomes occur when the care is appropriate to the patient's needs. Health care implemented according to standards will prevent negative outcomes for the patient. Thus, outcome standards describe the absence of negative outcomes as well as the presence of positive outcomes.

Outcome standards should be developed for all procedures and units of care. Chapter 3 explains how to write outcome standards related to patient satisfaction, procedures, and units of care. Chapter 4 describes how to write outcome standards for interdisciplinary units of care.

SUMMARY

The first five chapters explain the method for writing standards that has been developed over 20 years of research. After you learn this method, you will be able to write the standards for a procedure/unit of care in 30 minutes or less.

With a little practice you will begin to intertwine the steps of the method. For example, when writing the process standards for a procedure/unit of care you may find that an outcome or an additional goal may come to mind. This thought may prompt you to think of additional interventions/observations that will link the goals and patient outcomes together.

After standards are written, they must go through the process of validation. The description of this process is explained in chapters 6 and 7.

Then you are ready to implement the standards. Chapter 8 explores the implementation of standards.

Now select a chapter to begin writing meaningful standards.

NOTES

1. Donabedian, A. "Criteria and standards for quality assessment and monitoring." *Quality Review Bulletin, 12* (3), pp. 99–108, 1986.
2. Ibid.
3. Ibid.

2

Writing Process Standards

Process standards define the quality of nursing care. All procedures and units of care require process standards. A **process standard** defines what nursing care must be done to guarantee positive outcomes. Process standards in a procedure are the steps in a procedure that must be implemented. The process standards within a unit of care are the interventions, observations, and principles that must be followed to ensure positive outcomes for a patient. The purposes of process standards are to:

- Provide a consistent approach to each patient
- Ensure that valid interventions are implemented in nursing care
- Assure that all nurses implementing the standards understand them
- Reduce the time required to plan nursing care
- Provide the framework for nurses to easily individualize care for each patient

This chapter has been designed to explain the method for writing process standards. The first section contains the method for writing standards for a nursing procedure. Developing process standards for units of care are the topics for sections 2 and 3. Section 4 defines the differences between a process standard and a rationale or a suggestion. Each section of this chapter can be studied independently of the others. Additional examples of process standards will be found in the appendix.

SECTION 1

Writing Process Standards for Procedures

All procedures should contain process standards to ensure the goals of the procedure will be met. Thus, the patient will not experience preventable complications or unnecessary discomfort during the implementation of the procedure. A **procedure** contains the process and outcome standards that define what must be done to:

- Alter the patient's internal or external environment for the patient's benefit
- Prevent complications
- Involve the family in assisting the patient in coping with or preventing health problems
- Increase the psychological or physiological comfort of the patient
- Change the patient's environment

Examples of procedures include:

- Care of a patient with an indwelling urinary catheter
- Discharge of a patient
- Admitting a patient to the seclusion room
- Assisting the patient with patient-controlled analgesia
- Wet to dry dressing
- Nursing care of a neonate on a ventilator
- Nursing care of a child in a croupette

Before proceeding with the study of the method for writing process standards for a procedure, stop and ask yourself:

- Do I understand the definition of a nursing procedure?

If the answer is "yes," go on to the next part of this section. If the answer is "no," reread the definition of a nursing procedure at the beginning of the section.

METHOD

The eight steps in writing process standards for a procedure are:

1. Select a procedure.
2. List the goals of the procedure.
3. Identify the steps in the procedure essential in achieving the goals.
4. List pertinent observations.
5. Specify when each of the essential steps and observations in the procedure needs to be done.
6. Combine the process standards in a logical order.
7. Eliminate suggestions and rationale from the standards you have written.
8. Establish the validity of the process standards.

When you complete the last step, you will have process standards ready for implementation.

If you have already developed outcome standards for the procedure, begin with step 3.

STEP 1
Identify the Procedure

Select the nursing procedure for which you need to write standards. The example that will illustrate the method is the nursing procedure *Nursing Care of the Patient Receiving Intermittent Tube Feedings.*

STEP 2
Identify the Goals of the Procedure

A **goal** is an explicit statement describing exactly what you plan to accomplish with your nursing care. Goals should describe the results of nursing care in relation to the effect upon the patient, the patient's family or an improvement in the patient's environment. Goals include prevention of negative outcomes as well as positive outcomes. As you think about the reasons for implementing this procedure, ask yourself:

- What are the intended results of this procedure?
- Why is this procedure usually implemented?
- What complications can I prevent for the patient while administering this nursing procedure?

The goals for this procedure are:

1. The patient will understand the procedure.
2. The patient will not experience aspiration during or after the feeding.
3. The patient will tolerate the feeding.
4. The patient will not experience nausea, vomiting, or diarrhea.
5. The patient will be comfortable before, during, and after the feedings.

Note: When the goals are individualized for a specific patient, the exact date for the achievement of each goal must be defined in terms of whether the procedure is implemented over a period of time or needs to be repeated to achieve the goal.

After identifying all the goals of the procedure, proceed to step 3.

STEP 3
Identify the Steps in the Procedure Essential in Achieving the Goals

For each goal ask yourself:

- What must I do when implementing the procedure to meet this goal?
- What steps in the procedure are essential in meeting this goal?
- What procedures are essential in preventing negative outcomes for the patient?
- What steps must be implemented to provide for the patient's comfort during the procedure?
- Have all the legal safeguards for the patient been included?

The answers to these questions are the essential steps in this procedure.

For Goal 1, *the patient will understand the procedure,* the essential step in the procedure is:

- Explain the procedure to the patient.

For Goal 2, *the patient will not experience aspiration during or after the feeding,* the essential steps in the procedure are:

- Position the patient in high Fowler's.

- Check tube for correct position.

For Goal 3, *the patient will tolerate his/her feedings*, the essential steps in the procedure are:

- The feeding is room temperature.
- Aspirate stomach contents for residual feeding.
- Clear the air from the tubing.
- Maintain feeding flow at the prescribed rate.
- Irrigate the feeding tube with 30–50cc tap water (room temperature).

For Goal 4, *the patient will not experience nausea, vomiting, or diarrhea,* the essential steps in the procedure are:

- If the equipment is not clean or has an odor, use new equipment.
- Clean the bag and tubing well.
- Change equipment.

For Goal 5, *the patient will be comfortable before, during, and after the feedings*, the essential steps in the procedure are:

- Provide for the patient's physical comfort.
- Provide privacy.
- Reassure the patient.
- Provide rest periods.
- Provide oral hygiene.

After you have identified all of the required steps in the procedure, review all of the goals and answer this question:

- Have I included all the legal safeguards for the patient?

If your answer is "yes," go on to the next step. If your answer is "no," write additional nursing actions until all the safeguards have been included. Then proceed to step 4.

STEP 4
List Pertinent Observations

Now, review the goals of the procedure and ask yourself:

- What observations must I make to monitor the patient's responses to this procedure?

For *Nursing Care of the Patient Receiving Intermittent Tube Feedings*, the observations to be made are:

- Observe for aspiration.
- Observe for nausea, vomiting, and diarrhea.
- Observe the condition of the equipment.
- Ask the patient if the patient understands the procedure.

STEP 5
Specify When Each of the Essential Steps in the Procedure Needs to Be Done

Examine each of the steps in the procedure and specify when it needs to be done. Process standards must have an action and a *frequency or time* when they are done unless the time is implied in the statement of the action.

Before the feeding:

- Explain the procedure to the patient.
- Provide privacy.
- Position patient in high Fowler's unless contraindicated.
- Provide for the patient's physical comfort.
- Use new equipment if the feeding equipment is not clean or has an odor.
- Ensure the feeding is room temperature.
- Check the tube for correct position.
- Aspirate stomach contents for residual feeding. (If 50cc or less, replace aspirant and give feeding. If 50–100cc, return aspirant and hold feeding.)
- Clear the air from the tubing.

During the feeding:

- Maintain feeding flow at the prescribed rate.
- Reassure the patient PRN.
- Keep the patient in high Fowler's position, unless contraindicated. Observe for aspiration.

After the feeding:

- Keep the patient in high Fowler's position for 30 minutes.
- Irrigate the feeding tube with 30–50cc tap water (room temperature).

- If feeding is withheld, check *in one hour*. If greater than 100cc, return aspirant and withhold feeding. If unable to feed, notify the physician.
- Clean the bag and tubing well.
- Provide oral hygiene *every 4 hours and PRN*.
- Change equipment *every 24 hours.*
- Provide rest periods *between feedings.*

Note: There are some clinical settings where the equipment does not have to be changed every 24 hours because of the method used to clean the equipment.

Observations also require a *frequency or time* when they are done unless the time is implied in the statement of the observation. Now review the essential observations and identify when each of them must be done. The italicized portion of the observation clarifies when it should be done.

- Observe the condition of the equipment *before the feeding begins*.
- Ask the patient if he or she understands the procedure *before it begins*.
- Observe for aspiration *during or after the feeding.*
- Observe for nausea, vomiting, and diarrhea *after the feeding.*

After you have specified the time frame for those steps requiring one, you have completed writing a process standard.

STEP 6
Combine the Process Standards in a Logical Order

The completed procedure includes the goals and lists the process standards in the order that nurses will implement them.

Procedure

Nursing Care of a Patient Receiving Intermittent Tube Feedings

Goals

1. The patient will understand the procedure.
2. The patient will not experience aspiration during or after the feeding.
3. The patient will tolerate the feeding.
4. The patient will not experience nausea, vomiting, or diarrhea from contaminated feedings.

5. The patient will be comfortable before, during, and after the feedings.

Note: When the goals are individualized for a specific patient, the exact date for the achievement of the goal must be defined in terms of whether the procedure is implemented over a period of time or needs to be repeated to achieve the goals of the procedure.

Process Standards

Before the feeding:

1. Explain the procedure to the patient
2. Provide privacy.
3. Ask the patient if he or she understands the procedure.
4. Position patient in high Fowler's, unless contraindicated.
5. Provide for the patient's physical comfort.
6. Observe the condition of the feeding equipment.
7. Use new equipment if the feeding equipment is not clean or has an odor.
8. Ensure the feeding is room temperature.
9. Check the tube for correct position.
10. Aspirate stomach contents for residual feeding. (If 50cc or less, replace aspirant and give feeding. If 50–100cc, return aspirant and hold feeding.)
11. Clear the air from the tubing.

During the feeding:

12. Maintain feeding flow at the prescribed rate.
13. Reassure the patient PRN.
14. Keep the patient in high Fowler's position unless contraindicated.
15. Observe for aspiration.

After the feeding:

16. Keep the patient in high Fowler's position for 30 minutes unless contraindicated.
17. Observe for aspiration.
18. Irrigate the feeding tube with 30–50cc of tap water (room temperature) after the feeding.

by which the concept can be defined. Through experience and research we identify the characteristics of events, patients, and situations that are shared by others and therefore are examples of a particular concept. Recognizing that a new patient, event, or situation is an example of an already defined concept, nurses can generalize past experience to the new event, situation, or patient.

We can define nursing care using concepts because every patient having certain characteristics or experiencing a particular situation/event will require similar nursing care. An example of a concept is *Anxiety*. Many patients experience anxiety regardless of their other problems or needs. Thus, the process standards written for the care of one anxious patient are applicable to other anxious patients.

Concepts of various levels of generalizability can be used to develop units of care. The degree of generality of a concept is its degree of applicability. For example, the concept *Immobilization* is pertinent to the nursing care of many patients. Other examples of concepts with broad applicability are *Pain, Grieving, Family, Postoperative Care, Universal Precautions*, and each stage in *Growth and Development*.

METHOD

The nine steps in writing process standards for a concept unit of care are:

1. Define the unit of care.
2. Specify the time frame.
3. Identify the goals of nursing care.
4. List the interventions that will meet the goals.
5. Identify the observations related to the patient's responses and the patient's progress.
6. Specify when each intervention and observation needs to be done.
7. Combine the process standards in a logical order.
8. Eliminate suggestions and rationale from the process standards you have written.
9. Establish the validity of the process standards.

When you complete the last step, you will have process standards that are ready for implementation. If you have already developed outcome standards for the unit of care, begin with step 4.

STEP 1
Define the Unit of Care

There is often more than one way to define a concept. An **operational definition of a concept** contains a description of the concept written in a way that is clear to the nurses who are developing and implementing the standards. You should define the concept so that the goals of the unit of care are readily discernible. To test the operational definition, try to write the goals of the nursing care of the patient. If you are unable to identify the goals, the operational definition must be clarified. For example, an operational definition of the concept *Immobilization* is the unavoidable restriction or limitation of a patient so that she is not up, out of bed, and active more than 3 hours a day.

STEP 2
Specify the Time Frame

Every unit of care requires a time frame. Nursing care must be pertinent to the needs of the patient as the patient moves along the health-illness- health continuum. For nursing care to be appropriate as the patient's needs change, you have to develop a unit of care for each time period during which a change is required in the patient's nursing care. For example, a patient after abdominal surgery will require different interventions and observations when experiencing absent bowel sounds as compared to when the patient has active bowel sounds.

STEP 3
Identify the Goals of Nursing Care

After the time frame of the concept has been defined, the goals of nursing care can be specified. Goals enable you to identify pertinent interventions for the unit of care. A **goal** is an explicit statement describing exactly what you plan to accomplish with your nursing care. To identify the goals related to a concept, think about the nursing care that is appropriate for a patient described in the concept. Ask yourself:

- What nursing care is appropriate for a patient experiencing this concept?

A primary focus of nursing care for the patient experiencing the example concept *Immobility* is the prevention of complications that can arise from the effects of the immobilization. One of the potential complications of immobility is pneumonia. Some of the goals for the immobilized patient are:

- The patient will not experience stasis of secretions and hypostatic pneumonia.
- The patient will experience maximal chest expansion and respiratory excursion.

Note: When the goals are individualized for a specific patient, the exact date for the achievement of the goal must be defined.

After you have identified the goals, proceed to step 4.

STEP 4
List the Interventions That Will Meet the Goals

Now identify the interventions essential to meeting each of the goals you have defined. You may want to review the definition of an intervention in section 1 of this chapter. For each goal, ask yourself:

- What interventions must be implemented to meet this goal?

For example, consider this goal: *The patient will not experience stasis of secretions and hypostatic pneumonia:*

- What can the nurse do to prevent stasis of secretions and pneumonia?

The following interventions are examples of answers to that question:

- Position patient to maintain a patent airway and for optimal breathing.
- Encourage deep breathing and coughing unless contraindicated.
- Turn and reposition the patient unless contraindicated.

Now identify the interventions related to this goal: *The patient will experience maximal chest expansion and respiratory excursion:*

- Position patient to maintain a patent airway and for optimal breathing.
- Encourage deep breathing and coughing unless contraindicated.

Note: There is overlap between the interventions for the goals in this example, demonstrating that the goals are related.

Before proceeding, review the interventions you have written with the goals to ensure that you have not omitted any interventions. When you have identified all the interventions pertinent to each goal, proceed to step 5.

STEP 5
Identify the Observations Related to the Patient's Responses and the Patient's Progress

Now you need to identify the observations that must be made to determine the patient's responses to the interventions and the patient's progress. Examine each intervention and ask yourself:

- What observations must I make to monitor the patient's responses to each intervention?

Examine each goal and ask yourself:

- What do I need to monitor to identify the patient's progress toward the goals/outcome standards?

The following observations are answers to these questions:

- Auscultate all lobes of both lungs. Report abnormals to the physician or respiratory therapist.
- Observe the character of the respirations. Report changes to the physician or respiratory therapist.
- Observe the character of the sputum. Report changes to the physician or respiratory therapist.

STEP 6
Specify When Each Intervention/ Observation Needs to be Done

After you have identified the essential interventions/observations, you need to specify when each should be done. Think about each intervention and answer this question:

- How frequently does this intervention need to be done to achieve the goals/outcome standards?

For some goals, this question is more appropriate:

- When does this intervention need to be done to meet the goals/outcome standards?

This question may also be useful:

- How long must this intervention be done to achieve the goals/outcome standards ?

Following is a list of interventions, with times of implementation, for *nursing care of a patient who is immobilized with a potential for pneumonia:*

- Position patient to maintain a patent airway and for optimal breathing *at all times*.
- Encourage deep breathing and coughing *every hour* when awake unless contraindicated.
- Turn and reposition the patient *every 2 hours* unless contraindicated.

After you have specified when each of the interventions must be done to achieve the goals, you have developed process standards for the interventions. Now ask the following questions about each observation:

- *How frequently* does each observation need to be made in order to determine the patient's responses to each intervention and the patient's progress toward the goals/outcome standards?
- *How long* must each observation be done in order to determine the patient's responses to each intervention and the patient's progress toward the goals/outcome standards?
- *When* should each observation be made in order to determine the patient's responses to each intervention and the patient's progress toward the goals/outcome standards?

Read each observation and specify when each must be done. If you are not sure when an observation should be done, review when the intervention related to that observation is being implemented.

Consider also when it is feasible to make the observations. For example, if you are going to implement an intervention concerning a particular part of the patient's body and an observation needs to be made related to that part of the body, plan to perform the observation and intervention at the same time; for example, as the nurse does oral hygiene, observations related to the condition of the mouth and lips can be made.

The times for the observations for *nursing care of the patient who is immobilized with the potential for pneumonia* are specified here:

- Auscultate all lobes of both lungs *every 4 hours*. Report abnormals to the physician or respiratory therapist.
- Observe the character of the respirations *every 4 hours*. Report changes to the physician or respiratory therapist.
- Observe the character of the sputum *every 4 hours*. Report changes to the physician or respiratory therapist.

After you have specified a time for the implementation of the observations, you have developed process standards. After completing this step, go on to step 7.

STEP 7
Combine the Process Standards in a Logical Order

The finished unit of care identifies the unit of care, lists its goals, and combines the process standards in a way nurses will implement them. Now, combine the standards in a way most useful to the nurses implementing the standards. For some units of care, listing the standards in the chronological order of their implementation is the best way to combine them. For other units of care, because several standards need to be implemented concurrently, these standards are grouped together.

Unit of Care

Potential for Pneumonia

Goals

1. The patient will not experience atelectasis, stasis of secretions, and hypostatic pneumonia.
2. The patient will experience maximal chest expansion and respiratory excursion.

Note: When the goals are individualized for a specific patient, the exact date for the achievement of each goal must be defined.

Process Standards

1. Position patient to maintain a patent airway and optimal breathing at all times.
2. Encourage deep breathing and coughing (staged or cascade) qh when awake, unless contraindicated.
3. Turn and reposition the patient q2h unless contraindicated.
4. Auscultate all lobes of both lungs q4h. Report abnormals to the physician or respiratory therapist.
5. Observe the character of the respirations q4h. Report changes to the physician or respiratory therapist.
6. Observe the character of the sputum q4h. Report changes to the physician or respiratory therapist.

STEP 8
Eliminate Suggestions and Rationale from the Process Standards You Have Written

Suggestions and rationale are sometimes mistakenly identified as process standards. Read section 4 of this chapter to determine whether any process standards you have written are really suggestions or rationales. Eliminate any suggestions and statements of rationale from your list of process standards. Then go on to step 9.

STEP 9
Establish the Validity of the Process Standards

Although you have developed process standards, they are not ready for implementation. Refer to chapter 5 to establish the validity of the process standards you have written.

You have completed the section on how to write process standards for a concept unit of care. Now you may proceed to the next section, "Writing Process Standards for a Nursing Diagnosis, Health Problem, or Patient Care Need Unit of Care." Or you may want to read "Writing Outcome Standards for a Concept Unit of Care" in section 4 of chapter 3.

SECTION 3

Writing Process Standards for a Nursing Diagnosis, Health Problem, or Patient Care Need Unit of Care

It is essential that nurses implementing nursing care can relate the standards to the titles of the units of care or they will not be used in planning care. Process standards need to be written for a unit of care for patients with a nursing diagnosis, health problem, or need that can be used to individualize nursing care for these patients, yet provide a consistent quality of care. Although nursing diagnosis is the most frequently used style of titling units of care, there are some patient care needs and health problems that are not easily written as nursing diagnoses. And, not all nurses understand how to implement the nursing diagnosis framework. Thus, some of the units of care may need to be written as health problems or patient care needs. If nursing diagnosis is a requirement of accrediting agencies, those nurses who understand this approach can write the titles of the units of care as nursing diagnoses.

There are several definitions of nursing diagnosis. The one most recently accepted at the Ninth Conference of the North American Nursing Diagnosis Association is that **nursing diagnosis** is a clinical judgment about individual, family, or community responses to actual or potential health problems/life processes.[1] A nursing diagnosis provides the basis for the selection of nursing interventions to achieve outcomes for which the nurse is accountable. An example of a nursing diagnosis is *Sleep Pattern Disturbance.*[2]

A **health problem** or **patient care need** can be defined as a collection of signs and symptoms that, taken together, constitute a picture of ill health or health care required by the patient. The patient care need or problem is expressed in a word or phrase that triggers in the mind of the nurse a picture of the patient care need or problem and the nursing care pertinent to its resolution. An example of a patient care need is the *Need for Sleep*. This need can also be stated as a health problem, *Insomnia*.

As you decide what names should be used to title units of care, review the titles of the units of care on the care plans being designed for patients in your agency. Also, review the legal and accrediting requirements for your agency to determine if there are specific requirements for labeling units of care. This information as well as the nurses' preferences will assist you in your identification of the labels for the units of care.

METHOD

The nine steps in writing process standards for a nursing diagnosis, health problem, or patient care need unit of care are:

1. Define the unit of care.
2. Specify the time frame.
3. Identify the goals of nursing care.
4. List the interventions that will meet the goals.
5. Identify the observations related to the patient's responses and the patient's progress.
6. Specify when each intervention and observation needs to be done.
7. Combine the process standards in a logical order.
8. Eliminate suggestions and rationale from the process standards you have written.

9. Establish the validity of the process standards.

STEP 1
Define the Unit of Care

A definition of the nursing diagnosis, health problem, or patient care need is usually required by those nurses developing and implementing the process standards for the unit of nursing care. The unit of care must be defined in such a way that those nurses implementing the standards will have the same mental picture of the unit of care as those nurses writing the standards. To test the operational definition, try to write the goals of the nursing care for the patient. If you are unable to define the goals, revise the operational definition.

The example unit of care can be described as a nursing diagnosis, *Fluid Volume Deficit*.[3] It can also be defined as *Dehydration* (health problem) or as the patient care *Need for Fluid Volume*. Regardless of the title for this unit of care, the operational definition that can be used for writing standards is that *the patient is experiencing symptoms from a significant fluid loss from her body*. After you have defined the unit of care, proceed to step 2.

STEP 2
Specify the Time Frame

Every unit of care has a time frame. The time frame for the nursing care of the patient experiencing a loss of body fluid is implied in the title of this unit of care. If you decide to create two units of care for the patient's decrease in body fluid, the time frame of one of these units of care could be defined as from extreme fluid loss until the fluid balance is beginning to be restored. The time frame for the second unit of care could be defined from the beginning restoration of fluid balance until the patient is well enough to be discharged from the health agency and the patient can describe how to prevent this problem from reoccurring. To identify whether a time frame is needed for a unit of care, ask yourself:

- At what identifiable time periods will the patient require a different unit of care?

- When must I change the nursing care as the patient's health status changes?

In our example, the time frame for the unit of care *Fluid Volume Deficit, Dehydration*, or *Need for Fluid Volume* is defined in the title. The time frame is when the patient is experiencing a decrease in body fluids that is affecting the patient's homeostasis. After you have considered a time frame for this unit of care, proceed to step 3.

STEP 3
Identify the Goals of Nursing Care

After the time frame of the nursing diagnosis (or health problem or need) has been defined, the goals of nursing care can be specified. Goals enable you to identify pertinent interventions for the unit of care. A **goal** is an explicit statement describing exactly what you plan to accomplish with your nursing care. To identify the goals related to a nursing diagnosis, health problem, or need, think about the nursing care that is appropriate for a patient described in the nursing diagnosis. Ask yourself:

- What nursing care is appropriate for a patient experiencing this nursing diagnosis/health problem/patient care need?

The goals for this unit of care are:

- The patient's level of hydration will improve.
- The patient will be comfortable.
- The patient's family will be kept informed of the patient's status.
- Before discharge, the patient will be able to describe how to prevent a decreased level of hydration. (Content standards related to this goal are in the appendix.)
- The patient will not experience fluid overload.

Note: When the goals are individualized for a specific patient, the exact date for the achievement of the goal must be defined.

After you have identified the goals, proceed to step 4.

STEP 4
List the Interventions That Will Meet the Goals

Now identify the interventions essential to meeting each of the goals you have defined. You may want to review the definition of an intervention in section 1 of this chapter. For each goal, ask yourself:

- What interventions must be implemented to meet this goal?

Let's study the first goal: *The patient's level of hydration will improve.*

- What can nurses do to improve the patient's level of hydration?

The following interventions are examples of answers to that question:

- Encourage fluid intake to _____cc per hour:
- Infuse parenteral fluid intake as ordered.

Note: Amount of intake is based on the patient's need as well as the patient's ability to assimilate fluids.

Now, let's examine the second goal: *The patient will be comfortable.* Ask yourself:

- What interventions can provide comfort for the patient who is experiencing fluid volume loss?

These interventions are the answers to that question:

- Assist the patient with activities of daily living as needed.
- Increase the patient's feeling of warmth as needed:
  - Adjust the room temperature.
  - Add warm but lightweight clothing as needed by the patient for comfort.
- Provide emotional support while giving care.

Note: If the patient is on bedrest, *Immobilization* will also be required.

Now identify the interventions related to this goal: *The patient's family will be kept informed of the patient's status.*

- Inform one member of the patient's family concerning the patient's status every eight hours and PRN. (This family member is identified by the patient as her representative.)

Note: If you have a unit of care related to the needs of the family, this intervention should be placed in that unit of care.

Lastly, identify the interventions related to this goal: *The patient will not experience fluid overload.*

- Encourage fluid intake to _____cc per hour.
- Infuse parenteral fluid intake as ordered.

Note: Amount of intake is based on the patient's need as well as the patient's ability to assimilate fluids.

There is an obvious overlap in the interventions related to the goals in this example. The overlap demonstrates that the goals are related. Before proceeding compare the interventions you have written with the goals to ensure that you have not omitted any interventions. When you have identified all of the interventions pertinent to each goal, proceed to step 5.

STEP 5
Identify the Observations Related to the Patient's Responses and the Patient's Progress

Now you need to identify the observations that must be made to determine the patient's responses to the interventions and the patient's progress. Examine each intervention and ask yourself:

- What observations must I make to monitor the patient's responses to this intervention?

Now, examine each goal and ask yourself:

- What do I need to monitor to identify the patient's progress toward this goal/outcome standard?

The following observations are answers to these questions:

- Observe the patient's level of hydration:*
   a. Skin turgor
   b. Dryness of the skin and mucous membranes
   c. Specific gravity of the urine
   d. Pulse-quality and rate
- Monitor intake and output.*
- Weigh patient.*
- Monitor lab results.*
- Observe the patient's level of consciousness.*
- Observe for fluid overload: rapid weight gain, shortness of breath.
- Observe for verbal and nonverbal indications of the patient's ability to do the activities of daily living.
- Observe for the patient's level of comfort with the temperature of the room.

*If significant changes occur, notify the physician.

STEP 6
Specify When Each Intervention and
Observation Needs to be Done

After you have identified the essential interventions and observations, you need to specify when each should be done. Think about each intervention and answer this question:

- *How frequently* does this intervention need to be done to achieve the goals/outcome standards?

For some goals, this question is more appropriate:

- *When* does this intervention need to be done to meet the goals/outcome standards?

This question may also be useful:

- *How long* must this intervention be done to achieve the goals/outcome standards?

Following is a list of interventions, with times of implementation, for the nursing care of a patient with a loss of fluid volume:

- Encourage fluid intake to _____cc *per hour.*
- Infuse parenteral fluid intake *as ordered.*
- Assist the patient with Activities of Daily Living *as needed.*
- Increase the patient's feeling of warmth *as needed:*
  - Adjust the room temperature *PRN.*
  - Add warm but lightweight clothing *as needed* by the patient for comfort.
- Provide emotional support *while giving care.*
- Inform one member of the patient's family concerning the patient's status *every 8 hours.*

An hourly time was not specified for several of the interventions. Data must be gathered before the frequency of these interventions can be determined for each patient. After you have specified when each of the interventions must be done to achieve the goals, you have developed process standards for the interventions.

Now ask the following questions about each observation:

- *How frequently* does each observation need to be made in order to determine the patient's responses to each intervention and the patient's progress toward the goals/outcome standards?

- *How long* must each observation be done in order to determine the patient's responses to each intervention and the patient's progress toward the goals/outcome standards?

- *When* should each observation be made in order to determine the patient's responses to each intervention and the patient's progress toward the goals/outcome standards?

Read each observation and specify when each must be done. If you are not sure when an observation should be done, review when the intervention related to that observation is being implemented.

Consider also when it is feasible to make the observations. For example, if you are going to implement an intervention concerning a particular part of the patient's body and an observation needs to be made related to that part of the patient's body, plan to perform the observation and intervention at the same time; for example, as the nurse does oral hygiene, observations related to the condition of the mouth and lips can be made.

The times for the observations are specified below:

- Observe the patient's level of hydration *every 2 hours.**
  a. Skin turgor
  b. Dryness of the skin and mucous membranes
  c. Specific gravity of the urine
  d. Pulse-quality and rate

- Monitor intake and output *every hour.**
- Weigh patient *daily.**
- Monitor lab results *as they are available.**
- Observe the patient's level of consciousness *every 2 hours.**
- Observe for fluid overload: rapid weight gain, shortness of breath, increased blood pressure *every hour.**
- Observe for verbal and nonverbal indications of the patient's ability to do the activities of daily living *while giving care.*
- Observe for the patient's level of comfort with the temperature of the room *while giving care.*

*If significant changes occur, notify the physician.

The observations related to lab results cannot be more specific than "when the results are available," unless a frequency for obtaining the lab samples related to the observations is specified.

After you have specified a time for the implementation of the observations, you have developed process standards. After completing this step, go on to step 7.

STEP 7
Combine the Process Standards in a Logical Order

The finished unit of care identifies the unit of care, lists its goals, and combines the process standards in a way nurses will implement them. There are various ways to combine standards for a unit of care. If several standards need to be implemented concurrently, they can be grouped. Listing the standards in the chronological order of their use is another technique for combining standards. Before beginning this step, think about how the standards you have written will be implemented. A suggested way to combine the standards for this unit of care is presented below.

Unit of Care

Nursing Diagnosis: Fluid Volume Deficit
Health Problem: Dehydration
Patient Care Need: Need for Fluid Volume

Goals

1. The patient's level of hydration will improve.
2. The patient will be comfortable.
3. The patient's family will be kept informed of the patient's status.
4. Before discharge, the patient will be able to describe how to prevent a decreased level of hydration. (Content standards for this goal are in the appendix.)
5. The patient will not experience fluid overload.

Note: When the goals are individualized for a specific patient, the exact date for the achievement of the goal must be defined.

Process Standards

1. Encourage fluid intake to _____cc per hour.
2. Infuse parenteral fluid intake as ordered.
3. Monitor intake and output qh.*
4. Observe for fluid overload: rapid weight gain, shortness of breath, increased blood pressure qh.*

5. Observe the patient's level of hydration q2h.*
   a. Skin turgor
   b. Dryness of the skin and mucous membranes
   c. Specific gravity of the urine
   d. Pulse-quality and rate
6. Observe the patient's level of consciousness q2h.*
7. Observe for verbal and nonverbal indications of the patient's ability to do the activities of daily living while giving care.
8. Assist the patient with Activities of Daily Living as needed.
9. Observe for the patient's level of comfort with the temperature of the room while giving care.
10. Increase the patient's feeling of warmth as needed:
    a. Adjust the room temperature PRN.
    b. Add warm but lightweight clothing as needed by the patient for comfort.
11. Provide emotional support while giving care.
12. Weigh patient daily.*
13. Monitor lab results as they are available.*
14. Inform one member of the patient's family concerning the patient's status q8h and PRN. (This family member is identified by the patient as her representative.)

*If significant changes occur, notify the physician.

STEP 8
Eliminate Suggestions and Rationale from the Process Standards You Have Written

Suggestions and rationale are sometimes mistakenly identified as process standards. Read section 4 of this chapter to determine whether any process standards you have written are really suggestions or rationales. Eliminate any suggestions and statements of rationale from your list of process standards. Then go on to step 9.

STEP 9
Establish the Validity of the Process Standards

Although you have developed process standards, they are not ready for implementation. Refer to chapter 5 to establish the validity of the process standards you have written.

SECTION 4

Suggestions and Rationale

Suggestions and rationale are frequently found with process standards in procedures/units of care. Although suggestions and rationale may provide useful information for the nurse, they should not be confused with process standards. This section explains how to recognize suggestions and rationale.

SUGGESTIONS

A **suggestion** is a technique proposed by a nurse for implementing the standards of a procedure/unit of care. As a nurse becomes experienced in the use of a specific procedure, that nurse usually develops an effective approach for implementing the standards related to the procedure.

Suggestions are very helpful, especially for practitioners who are just beginning to implement procedures. Suggestions are usually related to equipment and materials used by nurses, how they hold equipment and materials, positioning of the patient, how to attach tubes, dressings, and other items to the patient, and verbal approaches to the patient and family. For example, a patient can assume various positions for an ostomy irrigation, or the equipment can vary, especially in the home situation.

Process standards provide a nurse a chance to be innovative while ensuring quality nursing care. Suggestions have a limited usefulness. If any of the factors in a situation varies a little, a given suggestion may not apply. Therefore, if you write suggestions in procedures/units of care, be sure to:

- Separate the process standards from the suggestions and label the suggestions appropriately
- Write suggestions that do not violate the process standards

Now read through the process standards you have written for a nursing procedure/unit of care to ascertain whether you have written any suggestions instead of process standards. If so, revise the process standards, labeling the suggestions accordingly.

RATIONALE

A **rationale** is an explanation of *why* a process standard for a procedure/unit of care should be implemented. Statements of rationale are helpful to nurses who are learning why to implement procedures/units of care as defined by the process standards. Such rationale statements also help reorient nurses to the standards for procedures/units of care they have not implemented for a long time.

For example, a process standard for *Intravenous Catheters* is to change the line and the dressing on the wounds every 24 hours using strict asepsis. The rationale for this standard is *to minimize the risk of introducing infection into the wound*.

Although rationale can be very helpful to nurses, it should not be confused with process standards. One of the purposes of process standards is to review nursing care when a patient experiences a negative outcome. Rationale cannot be used for evaluation. A rationale can state why a process standard should be implemented but a rationale cannot define the quality of nursing care. Therefore rationales should not be labeled as process standards. If you include rationale with process standards for a procedure/unit of care, separate the rationale and label it appropriately.

Now examine each of the process standards you have written to determine whether any process statement is really a rationale. If so, revise the process standards accordingly.

SUMMARY

After studying this chapter, you can write process standards for nursing procedures/units of care. Before you can establish the validity of process standards, outcome standards must be written for the same procedure/ unit of care. So, if you have not read chapter 3, "Writing Outcome Standards," it is suggested that you study it at this time.

You may want to write content standards concerning documentation, reporting, or teaching related to the process standards you have written. If so, proceed to chapter 5.

NOTES

1. Carpenito, Lynda Juall. *Nursing diagnosis: Application to clinical practice* (4th ed.), p.6. New York: JB Lipincott and Co., 1992.

2. Ibid., p.776.

3. Ibid., p.379.

3

Writing Outcome Standards

The focus of this chapter is how to write outcome standards for procedures and units of care. To ensure quality in the care provided to the patient, **outcome standards** are used to evaluate the patient's response to therapy and nursing care and his progress toward the goals. It is essential that you write outcome standards for every procedure and unit of care.

This chapter is divided into five sections. Section 1 describes the types of outcomes and the components of an outcome standard. How to write outcome standards concerning patient satisfaction is described in section 2. Section 3 contains the method for writing outcome standards for procedures. The last two sections focus on developing outcome standards for the two common types of units of care. Writing outcome standards for the concept type is in section 4, and the method for writing outcome standards for the nursing diagnosis, health problem, and patient care need unit of care is in section 5.

Each section can be studied independently of the others. Before you begin to study the method of writing outcome standards, read sections 1 and 2 which set the stage for the other sections. In sections 3 through 5, the following method for writing outcomes is employed: First, an overview of the method is presented; then, each step in the method is explained in more detail using procedures and units of care with their associated outcome standards as examples to illustrate each step. Questions are provided to guide your writing. The purpose of this approach is to help you thoroughly understand the method. Now, begin the study of writing outcome standards with sections 1 and 2.

SECTION 1

Types and Components of Outcome Standards

Outcome standards define (a) the expected change in the patient's health status after he has received care, (b) the expected change in the patient's environment after care, and (c) the extent of the patient's satisfaction with his care. Both positive and negative outcomes can result from therapy and care. Positive outcomes occur when the therapy and care are appropriate to meet the needs of patients, and the patients do not experience preventable complications.

Outcomes need to be designed so health professionals receive information concerning the patient's progress toward the outcomes while the patient is experiencing therapy and care to prevent negative outcomes such as untoward effects of the therapy and care or complications. Thus, it is important not only to define the final positive outcomes of the therapy and care, but also what dimensions of the patient and his environment should be observed during the implementation of the plan of care that identify his responses to the therapy and care and the progress toward the goals.

TYPES OF POSITIVE OUTCOMES

The positive outcomes of nursing care can be classified according to eleven types:

1. An improvement in the health status of the patient
2. Maintenance of the patient's health status unaffected by the patient's problem
3. An increase in the patient's psychological or physiological comfort

4. An increase in the knowledge of the patient and/or family needed to prevent a health problem
5. An increase in the knowledge of the patient and/or family needed to cope with a health problem
6. An increase in the patient's ability to cope with or prevent a health problem
7. An increase in the ability of the patient and family to cope with a health crisis
8. Increased acceptance of the patient by the patient's family
9. Patient satisfaction with nursing care received
10. An improvement in the patient's environment
11. An increase in the family's psychological or physiological comfort

In the first eight types of outcomes, the patient's psychological or physiological health status is *as good or better than* before receiving health care. The ninth type defines the outcomes through the eyes of the consumer. Because the patient's satisfaction with the care affects many of the outcomes, outcome standards concerning *patient satisfaction* should be developed.

An important type of positive outcome is *improvement in the patient's environment*. Because of the tremendous effect of the environment on the patient's health status, outcome standards concerning the environment need to be written.

The last type of positive outcome is an increase in the family's comfort. Because the family can be a valuable resource and can provide support to the patient, increasing its comfort can assist the patient to experience positive outcomes. Also, in many situations the family becomes the "patient."

TYPES OF NEGATIVE OUTCOMES

The following are types of possible negative outcomes of nursing care:

1. Deterioration of the patient's health status
2. Failure to maintain the patient's health status unaffected by the patient's health problem
3. Inability of the patient to cope with or prevent a health problem
4. Lack of knowledge of the patient and/or family needed to prevent a health problem
5. Disability

6. Lack of knowledge of the patient and/or family needed to cope with a health problem
7. Inability of the patient and/or family to cope with a health crisis
8. Psychological or physiological discomfort for the patient
9. Complications
10. Prolonged illness
11. Unwarranted death
12. Patient dissatisfaction with nursing care
13. Lack of improvement or deterioration of the patient's environment
14. Decreased acceptance of the patient by the patient's family or significant others
15. Psychological or physiological discomfort of the family

Although nursing care alone cannot prevent every possible negative outcome, many negative outcomes can be prevented by excellent nursing care. Thus, the absence of negative outcomes is a good indicator of the quality of nursing care.

Now that you know what types of outcomes can occur after nursing care, the components of a good outcome standard will be presented.

COMPONENTS OF OUTCOME STANDARDS

An **outcome standard** is the specific expected change in the patient's health status and the patient's environment after care has been provided. There are three components of an outcome standard:

- The expected outcome
- When the outcome will occur
- How the outcome can be detected

These components are described in the subsections that follow.

The Expected Outcome

An essential component of every standard is the outcome expected after excellent care has been administered. The **expected outcome** is the specific description of the impact of care on the patient, the family, or the patient's environment after the plan of care has been implemented. An example of an expected outcome for every type of positive and negative outcome is listed below:

Types of Positive Outcome	*Examples of Expected Outcome*
1. Improved health status	Patient not experiencing urgency, frequency, and burning on urination.
2. Maintained health status	Patient's bowel pattern is the same.
3. Increased psychological and physiological comfort	Patient's nonverbal behavior indicates decreased anxiety.
4. Increase in the knowledge of the patient and/or family needed to prevent a health problem	Patient can explain how to prevent infections.
5. Increase in the knowledge of the patient and/or family needed to cope with a health problem	Patient/family can explain how to take the antibiotic prescribed for the patient.
6. Increase in the patient's ability to cope with or prevent a health problem	Patient is not having recurring renal calculi.
7. Patient and family able to cope with a health crisis	Family obtained information and needed care from community resources for a patient with Amyotrophic Lateral Sclerosis.
8. Increased acceptance of the patient by the family	Family developed a plan to modify the house and assist the patient with rehabilitation.
9. Patient satisfaction with care	Patient expressed satisfaction on obtaining community resources needed to deal with arthritis.
10. Improvement in the patient's environment	Elimination of poison oak in a young child's play yard.
11. An increase in the family's psychological or physiological discomfort	The family expressed relief after receiving frequent progress reports concerning a patient whose condition is unstable.

Types of Negative Outcomes	*Examples of Expected Outcomes*
1. Deterioration of the patient's health status	Patient's fever is decreasing.
2. Failure to maintain the patient's health status unaffected by health problem	Patient's blood sugar is within normal limits.

3. Inability of the patient to cope with or prevent a health problem

Patient can demonstrate how to change his colostomy bag and irrigate the colostomy.

4. Inability of the patient to prevent a health problem

Absence of recurring renal calculi

5. Disability

Absence of Parkinson-like symptoms (patient is not experiencing a side effect from the use of the drugs used to treat his depression).

6. Lack of knowledge of the patient and/or family needed to cope with a health problem

Patient and family demonstrate how to do peritoneal dialysis in the home.

7. Inability of the patient and/or family to cope with a health crisis

Family can demonstrate how to do CPR and obtain medical assistance for a patient with chronic heart disease.

8. Psychological or physiological discomfort for the patient

Patient is not vomiting after chemotherapy.

9. Complications

Absence of congestive heart failure

10. Prolonged illness

Mother is able to resume the care of her children.

11. Unwarranted death

Patient is able to do activities of daily living without assistance.

12. Patient dissatisfaction with nursing care

Patient and family received resources and information needed to care for terminally ill patient at home.

13. Deterioration of the patient's environment

Patient is able to work in a smokeless environment.

14. Decreased acceptance of the patient by the patient's family

Family joins groups associated with Alcoholics Anonymous to be supportive of the patient.

The preceding examples demonstrate two styles of writing outcome standards related to the prevention of negative outcomes. One style is to write the standard as a *positive outcome*. As you probably noticed, most of the negative outcomes are the opposites of the positive outcomes. If it is possible to write the outcome standard for the prevention of a negative outcome as a positive outcome, do so.

The other style is to place the words *absence* or *lack of* before the outcome that you want to prevent. An example of this method is the expected outcome for Negative Outcome Type 9, *absence of congestive heart failure*.

I have presented two ways of writing outcome standards related to negative outcomes because one way is not appropriate for all kinds of outcome standards. In summary, all outcome standards are written as explicit, positive statements concerning the outcome of nursing care.

When the Outcome Will Occur

The time dimension—that is, when an outcome should be apparent—must be included in all standards. The time dimension enables the staff observing the patient for the outcome to know when the outcome should be present. The appropriate time period for the achievement of results for one procedure or unit of care is different from others, depending on the length of time it takes to produce the outcome.

Consider, for example, this outcome standard: *"Within one hour after secretions were suctioned from the patient's tracheostomy tube, the patient will not experience anoxia or cardiac arrest."* In this example the time period specified was *within 1 hour*.

Another example of an outcome standard is: *Before and during the procedure the patient says he is comfortable.* By asking a direct question about the patient's comfort before and during the procedure you can ascertain if the outcome has been achieved. If it has not been achieved, you can initiate the appropriate interventions.

There are some clinical areas in which the patient remains such a short time the patient's status needs to be evaluated *just before* the patient is transferred or discharged. Examples of these clinical areas are:

- Operating Room
- Postanesthesia
- Delivery
- Emergency Department
- Outpatient Department
- Home Visit

Evaluation of care using outcome standards is necessary to assure that the patient's health status is adequate before he leaves the clinical area or when the staff completes a visit to a patient's home. When this isn't done, preventable complications can occur. For example, a patient required a tourniquet on his finger to remove a tumor from his finger. The staff did not observe the patient before he left the Operating Room to see that the tourniquet was removed. *He returned to the unit with the tourniquet still in place. Subsequently, he had to have his finger amputated.*

Another patient had a leg cast applied in the Emergency Department. *The patient was given crutches that were 3 inches too long for him. He fell upon leaving the Emergency Department.* If a staff member had used outcome standards to evaluate these patients' status before leaving the clinical areas, they would not have had preventable complications.

For some units of care that require longer than a few hours for the outcome to become evident, you need to think of a continuum of interim outcomes that are points in time when decisions need to be made related to the patient's plan of care to ensure that the patient will reach his defined positive outcomes on discharge.

An interim outcome is the *status of the patient or his environment while he is receiving care that identifies that he is moving toward the goals and is not experiencing any negative outcomes*. Thus, a patient may have several interim outcomes before he reaches the defined positive outcomes of his unit of care. These interim outcomes are evaluated at a point in time that will provide data about the status of the patient. These data will assist the staff in their updating of the plan of care so that the patient:

a. Will not experience preventable complications
b. Will progress toward the goals
c. Will experience a continuity of care when discharged from one health facility to another facility or to the community

For example, in acute care facilities the average length of stay for patients has decreased from 10 days to 3 days, yet the care and teaching needed by the patient has not significantly changed. Interim outcome standards become the outcome standards that staff members use for decision-making regarding the care and teaching that can be completed while the patient is in the acute care facility and what will need to be completed after discharge.

In order to send a referral to the appropriate community agency, the patient's progress toward the goals needs to be evaluated at least two days before discharge. When the length of stay is less than two days, such as after delivery of a baby, the patient's responses to therapy and health status need to be evaluated *before* the patient leaves the facility. Then a referral, if needed, can be completed.

Some interventions must be repeated over a period of days or weeks before a significant change in a patient's health status occurs. Because outcome standards are needed to monitor the effectiveness of interventions, interim outcome standards for long-term goals need to be developed to determine that the patient is making progress.

If the interim outcome standards are not achieved within the designated time limit, the interventions can be modified or replaced with other interventions. Staff cannot afford to wait for weeks, even in long-term care, to confirm whether their interventions are effective, because a patient may be delayed in recuperation or may incur complications as a result of an ineffective intervention.

A rule of thumb to use in deciding the time period appropriate for defining interim standards for long-term care is a week. If an intervention requires implementation for 3 weeks to achieve a goal, interim standards should be developed for the positive outcomes that can be expected weekly.

The following example illustrates interim outcome standards for the nursing care goal *to teach the patient how to care for his colostomy.* The outcome standard is *the patient can demonstrate the care of his colostomy.*

The interim outcomes are that the patient and/or family can:

- Apply the colostomy bag correctly
- Recognize when the bag needs to be changed
- Regulate diet for effective functioning of the colostomy
- Irrigate the colostomy safely
- Clean and care for the colostomy equipment
- Use of special equipment and supplies

For each of these outcomes, there is a sequence of more interim outcomes that, when met in the appropriate sequence, result in the attainment of the overall outcome standard.

Where can you find information to develop interim outcomes? Although they do not usually contain written standards as such, textbooks do contain information to assist you in identifying interim standards. Also, staff providing nursing care for a particular type of patient are a source of information about interim outcomes. After you have identified all the interim outcomes related to an overall outcome standard, ask yourself:

- How long does it usually take to meet this standard?

The answer will provide you with a time frame for each standard. The following example will show you how interim outcomes, when met in sequence, can assist the nurse in reaching the overall outcome standard. The outcome standard *the patient can demonstrate that he can apply the colostomy bag* has several interim outcomes.

Within 2 days after surgery, the patient will observe while the nurse provides care of the colostomy. (The italicized words define the time period when the expected outcome can be observed.)

Within the next 3 days, after observing the care, the patient can change the colostomy bag with assistance from the nurse. The patient can state the standards needed to change the bag.

Within 7 days of surgery, the patient changes the colostomy bag correctly. He can explain the foods he should eat and those he should avoid, and how to do a colostomy irrigation. He also can state where to obtain information, equipment, and the supplies he will need.

You probably noticed that when the patient has met all the interim standards in the appropriate sequence, he has successfully demonstrated the care of his colostomy. By writing interim standards for outcome standards requiring a long period of time for achievement of the outcome standards, you can assess the patient's progress at frequent intervals. When the patient is not making progress you can implement other interventions when needed.

But suppose the patient will be discharged in 4 days. The nurse may not be able to teach what was usually taught when the patient's stay was 7 days. Knowing this, the nurse would write an interim outcome for the patient's status 2 days after surgery. At this critical point the nurse can estimate, given his present conditon, what the patient may be able to learn with two more days' instruction and begin to develop a referral for the teaching that might need to be done by a community agency.

In summary, "when" the patient's status needs to be evaluated must be included in every outcome standard. Now proceed with "How the Outcome Can Be Detected."

How the Outcome Can Be Detected

A statement of how the outcome can be detected provides the necessary specificity to the description of the outcome. To develop this segment of the outcome standard, you need to write an exact description of the behavior of the patient or of the patient's environment that you expect to see when the outcome standard is met. The following is an example of an outcome standard for the procedure *Suction the Tracheostomy*: "absence of hypoxia with 1 hour after suctioning as indicated by *an absence of changes in mental state, dyspnea, increase in pulse and blood pressure, arrhythmias, and cyanosis.*" The italicized signs and symptoms describe how to detect hypoxia in the patient.

The following is an example of an outcome standard for the procedure *Nursing Care of the Patient Receiving Intermittent Tube Feedings: Before the procedure, the patient understands the procedure.* The statement *The patient, if alert and responsive, briefly describes the procedure, what will happen during the procedure, and when to call the nurse* further clarifies what is expected as an outcome standard for this procedure.

If every one of the staff implementing the standards can identify the specific outcomes described in the standards, this component does not need to be written. On the other hand, if you believe there will be staff who may be unfamiliar with the procedures to be implemented, the required specificity can be added to the outcome standards. *The rule of thumb is to make the outcomes as specific as necessary for every person who will be implementing or evaluating the care of the patient to understand the outcomes.* Thus, this component of the standard can be omitted or explained in great detail depending on the knowledge and experience of those implementing the standard.

SECTION 2
Writing Outcome Standards for Patient Satisfaction

It is important that you write outcome standards concerning patient satisfaction for every nursing procedure and unit of care. The patient is not able to evaluate all aspects of nursing care. Patients can, however, provide valuable feedback to nurses about their approach to patients and families. The nurses' approach to patients often affects the outcome of nursing care. Thus, including outcome standards concerning patient satisfaction is very important in providing nursing care of excellent quality.

METHOD

To write standards for patient satisfaction, ask yourself:

• What can the patient expect of me while receiving nursing care?

An example of this type of standard is *nurses willingly answered the questions you asked.* Another example is *nurses explained treatments and diagnostic tests in a way that was clear to you.*

In the examples, notice that the standard is written in a form of a statement that requires a patient to make a judgment about the nursing care.

This is done because only patients can determine whether nursing care met their expectations.

Standards concerning patient satisfaction also are written in some form of the past tense because the patient is asked if the nursing care described in the statement *was provided*. Thus, even though the statements in the examples describe the process of nursing care, they are outcome statements because the patient is asked to respond to the quality of the nursing care after he has experienced it.

Another question you can ask yourself when writing outcome standards for patient satisfaction is:

- What can the nurse do to assist the patient with or prevention of his health problems?

An example of an answer to this question is *the nurse listened to your problem*. Another example is *the nurses comforted you during painful tests or treatments*.

Family members are also patients of the nurse. Thus, outcome standards concerning patient satisfaction are not complete without including standards concerning the family.

To write patient satisfaction standards pertaining to family, ask yourself:

- What can I do to assist the patient's family while the patient is receiving nursing care?
- What can I do to assist the family to accept and help the patient?

The following statements are some examples of outcome statements concerning patient satisfaction:

- The nurses were kind to your family.
- The nurses helped your family understand your progress.
- The nurses explained to your family members how they can help you when you return home.
- The nurses answered the questions your family members asked about your nursing care.

In summary, the essential characteristics of outcome standards concerning patient satisfaction are:

1. The outcome is written as a statement describing the nurses' approach to the patient while administering care.
2. The standard is written as a statement or question that the patient can respond to in relation to experiences with nursing care.
3. The statement is written in the past tense.

If you wish to evaluate whether your patients are satisfied with their nursing care, list the outcome standards on a sheet of paper. Ask the patients to place a "yes" beside the standard if the nursing care standard was met or a "no" if the nursing care did not meet the standard.

Or, patients may be asked to indicate their satisfaction with the nursing care by placing a mark on a continuum. For example, the patient responds to the outcome standard *the nurses listened to your problem* by selecting a point on a continuum:

All of the time _____ **Never**

Now that you have completed sections 1 and 2, select any of the next three sections to begin writing outcome standards. Section 3 concerns outcome standards for procedures, while sections 4 and 5 relate to outcome standards for units of care.

SECTION 3
Writing Outcome Standards for Procedures

This section describes the method of writing outcome standards for a procedure. A **procedure** contains the process and outcome standards that define what must be done to:

- Alter the patient's internal or external environment for the patient's benefit

- Change the patient's environment

- Prevent complications

- Involve the family in assisting the patient in coping with or preventing a health problem

- Increase the psychological or physiological comfort of the patient

Outcome standards define the expected change in the patient's health status or environment after the procedure has been implemented. A procedure may contain multiple interventions, but its focus is a specific facet of a patient's care. The following are examples of titles of procedures:

- Colostomy Irrigation
- Safe Administration of Anticoagulants
- Nursing Care of a Patient with an Endotracheal Tube

- Assisting the Patient When Crutch Walking
- Continuous Monitoring of Systemic Arterial Pressure
- Obtaining a Sputum Culture
- Continuous Fetal Monitoring

Now, proceed to the method of writing outcome standards.

METHOD

The eight steps in writing outcome standards for a procedure are:

1. Identify the procedure.
2. Identify the goals of the procedure.
3. Identify the positive outcomes that are expected to occur.
4. Identify the negative outcomes that can be prevented.
5. Specify when you expect each outcome to occur.
6. Clarify the description of the expected outcomes.
7. Combine the outcome standards in a logical order.
8. Establish the validity of the outcome standards.

After you have completed step 8, you will have valid outcome standards that are ready for implementation. Now that you have read an overview of the method, you are ready to begin a more detailed study of each step.

STEP 1
Identify the Procedure

Select the procedure for which you need to write outcome standards. The example used to illustrate this method is the procedure *Nursing Care of a Patient Receiving Intermittent Tube Feedings.*

STEP 2
Identify the Goals of the Procedure

A **goal** is an explicit statement describing exactly what you plan to accomplish with your nursing care. You need to include goals for preventing negative outcomes as well as those that result in positive outcomes for the patient or the patient's family. As you think about the procedure, ask yourself:

- What can this procedure do for a patient?
- What complications can I prevent for the patient while administering this nursing procedure?

For the procedure *Nursing Care of a Patient Receiving Intermittent Tube Feedings*, the goals are:

- The patient will understand the procedure.
- The patient will not experience aspiration during or after the feeding.
- The patient will tolerate the feeding.
- The patient will not experience nausea, vomiting, or diarrhea.
- The patient will be comfortable before, during, and after the feedings.

Note: When the goals are individualized for a specific patient, the exact date for the achievement of each goal must be defined in terms of whether the procedure is implemented over a period of time or needs to be repeated to achieve the goals.

After identifying all the goals of the procedure, proceed to step 3.

STEP 3
Identify the Positive Outcomes That Are Expected to Occur

Before proceeding with this step, you may want to review "Types of Positive Outcomes" and "The Expected Outcome" in section 1 of this chapter. To identify the positive outcomes of a procedure, examine each procedure and ask:

- If this goal is met, what results can I expect?

The answer to this question will assist you in identifying one or more positive outcomes. For example, for the goal *the patient will understand the procedure*, the outcome is *the patient can describe the procedure and his participation in it.* This outcome is an example of Positive Outcome Type 3, increased psychological and physiological comfort.

For the goal *the patient will be comfortable before and during the feedings*, the outcome is *the patient says he is comfortable.* This outcome is another example of Positive Outcome Type 3.

For the goal *the patient will tolerate the feeding*, the outcome is *the patient ingests the feeding.* This outcome statement is an example of Positive Outcome Type 1, an improvement in the health status of the patient.

After you have identified all the positive outcomes for every goal of the procedure, go to step 4.

STEP 4
Identify the Negative Outcomes That Are Expected to Occur

Before proceeding with this step, you may want to review "Types of Negative Outcomes" in section 1 of this chapter.

By answering the following questions, you can identify the negative outcomes that can be prevented by implementing the goals of the procedure. For each goal, ask yourself:

- What negative outcomes can I prevent if this goal is met?
- If the nursing care related to this goal is not administered, what negative outcomes may occur?

Look at the following goals and try to identify the negative outcomes that can be avoided if the nursing care appropriate to these goals is administered. For example, for the goal *the patient will not experience aspiration during or after the feeding,* ask yourself:

- If this goal is met, what results would I expect?

The answer to this question is *absence of aspiration,* an example of Negative Outcome Type 9, *complications.*

All negative outcomes are written as positive statements to ensure clarity when used for evaluation. For example, if this outcome were written as *the patient experienced aspiration of the feeding during the procedure,* the answer "no" would indicate that the patient's care met the standard. Other outcomes for this evaluation might be stated such that a "no" answer would mean the patient was experiencing a complication. *Thus, all outcome standards should be written so that every "yes" in response to the standard means the patient experienced a positive outcome.*

For the goal *the patient will not experience complications,* the outcome is *the absence of diarrhea, nausea, and vomiting.* This outcome is an example of Negative Outcome Type 9, *complications.*

After you have identified all the negative outcomes related to the goals of the procedure and developed them into positive statements, study the next step.

STEP 5
Specify When You Expect Each Outcome to Occur

You may want to review "When the Outcome Will Occur" in section 1 of this chapter before proceeding with this step. Now examine each of the outcome statements you have written and ask yourself:

• When can I expect this outcome to occur?

Consider, for example, the outcome statement "absence of diarrhea, nausea, and vomiting *within six hours of the feeding*." The italicized portion of this outcome statement specifies when you can observe the outcome. This time frame requires the nurse to compare the patient's outcome to the patient's status before the feeding. If the patient experiences any of these problems as an outcome, the equipment may have been contaminated, the feeding was exposed to a warm room temperature for too long, the patient's electrolyte status is abnormal, or the patient has an unknown allergy to the feeding. In addition to calling the physician for medication to treat the symptoms, the nurse should and can explore the cause(s) of the problem.

The following outcomes are related to prevention type goals. When the procedure is done correctly, the outcome should be positive every time you observe the patient.

• There is an absence of aspiration *at all times* during or after the feeding.

• *At all times* during the procedure, the patient says that he is comfortable.

The phrase "at all times" defines when this outcome can be observed. If the nurses know that "at all times" is understood when reading these outcomes, you can omit the phrase from the outcomes.

Lastly, *"Before beginning the procedure*, the patient can describe the procedure and his participation in it" defines *when* you would ask the patient if he understood the procedure.

Note: When the outcomes are individualized for a specific patient, the exact date for the achievement of the outcome must be defined.

After you have specified in each statement when to look for the outcome, go on to step 6.

STEP 6
Clarify the Description of the Expected Outcomes

Before beginning this step, you may want to review "How the Outcome Can Be Detected" in section 1 of this chapter. Now examine the description of the outcome you wrote in steps 2 and 3. It is important to make the description of the outcome as detailed as is needed by those nurses implementing the nursing care related to the standard.

For example, consider the outcome statement "absence of aspiration during and after the feeding *as indicated by: noiseless respirations, absence of respiratory congestion, and the patient's ease in breathing."* If all the nurses who will be observing patients for this outcome demonstrate that they know the signs and symptoms of aspiration, the italicized portions of the outcome statement do not need to be included. If nurses are not knowledgeable about the specific observations to be made, however, this part of the outcome statement becomes extremely vital to the implementation of the standard.

The specification of the other outcome statements are written as follows:

- "The patient ingests the feeding, *as indicated by less than 50cc of feeding aspirated from the stomach before the next feeding is given."*

- "Absence of diarrhea, nausea, and vomiting after the feeding. If the patient experiences *any diarrhea, nausea and vomiting within six hours after the feeding,* the potential cause of it should be investigated by the nurse."

- "Before the procedure, the patient can describe the procedure and his participation in it, if alert and responsive. *The patient briefly describes the procedure, what will happen during the procedure, and when to call the nurse."*

Again, it is not essential to include the italicized words in the outcome standard if all nurses implementing the standard demonstrate they know these indicators. After each outcome statement has successfully gone through these first six steps in the method, it is an outcome standard. Now proceed to step 7.

STEP 7
Combine the Outcome Standards in a Logical Order

The completed procedure includes its title, lists its goals, and combines the outcome standards in a logical order. There are many ways to arrange the outcome standards you have written.

Because outcome standards are used to evaluate the quality of nursing care, they should be grouped to facilitate evaluation. Outcome standards can be grouped into those standards for which data are obtained from the patient and those for which data are obtained from the chart. Or, the outcome standards can be placed in chronological order in which the data would be collected. For this example, the outcomes are placed in chronological order.

Procedure

Nursing Care of a Patient Receiving Intermittent Tube Feedings

Goals

1. The patient will understand the procedure.
2. The patient will not experience aspiration during or after the feeding.
3. The patient will tolerate the feeding.
4. The patient will not experience nausea, vomiting, or diarrhea.
5. The patient will be comfortable before, during, and after the feedings.

Outcome Standards

1. Absence of aspiration during and after the feeding, as indicated by noiseless respirations, absence of respiratory congestion, and the patient's ease in breathing.
2. The patient ingests the feeding, as indicated by less than 50cc of feeding aspirated from the stomach before the next feeding is given.
3. Absence of diarrhea, nausea, and vomiting within 6 hours after the feeding.
4. Before the procedure, the patient can describe the procedure and his participation in it, if alert and responsive. The patient briefly describes the procedure, what will happen during the procedure, and when to call the nurse.
5. Before and during the procedure, the patient says he is comfortable.

Note: When the outcomes are individualized for a specific patient, the exact date for the achievement of the outcome must be defined in terms of whether the procedure is implemented over a period of time or needs to be repeated to achieve the goals of the procedure.

Now go on to step 8.

STEP 8
Establish the Validity of the Outcome Standards

Although you have written outcome standards, they are not ready to be implemented. Study chapter 5 to establish the validity of these standards.

SECTION 4

Writing Outcome Standards for a Concept Unit of Care

Concepts are very useful in developing units of care. A **concept** is a group of objects, events, or processes with common characteristics or attributes that define the concept. Concepts can assist you in the identification of the commonalities of nursing care of patients with various health problems. As a result of the evolution of nursing practice and research, the interventions essential to the care of one patient have been found to be applicable in the care of patients with other health problems and patient care needs. Recognizing that the nursing care of one patient is the same as another patient, you can generalize your past experience to the new clinical situations. Thus, concepts can facilitate the development of units of care by assisting in the organization of your thoughts about nursing care.

Concepts have different degrees of general applicability. Concepts with broad general applicability can assist you in developing units of care pertinent to the needs of patients in many settings. Examples of concepts with broad general applicability are *Immobilization*, *Peri-Operative Care*, *Spiritual Needs*, *Skin Integrity*, *Health Teaching*, and *Change in Body Image*.

There are other concepts that apply to fewer patients. For example, *Arterial Line Insertion Site Care* is appropriate for fewer patients than the concept, *Wound Care*. Other examples of concepts that are useful in planning nursing care for fewer groups of patients are: *Septic Shock*, *Hypertensive Crisis*, and *Long-Term Memory Loss*.

Concepts are very helpful in developing units of care because the concept can assist in creating a mental picture for the person writing the standards. A **unit of care** contains a cluster of process, content, and outcome standards that define nursing care required by a patient. When using concepts to develop units of care, you must define the concept so the nurse implementing the care can mentally visualize the same care for the patient as the nurse who developed the standard. For example, if you asked the nurse implementing the standards for *Potential for Urinary Tract Infection* to list the outcome standards for the *Potential for Urinary Tract Infection* unit of care, the outcome standards should agree with the written standards.

For example, an essential concept with broad general applicability is *Immobilization*. *Immobilization* is the prescribed or unavoidable restriction or limitation of a patient so that she is not up, out of bed, and active more than three hours a day. Immobilization has several subconcepts that need to be developed into units of care, such as *Potential for Urinary Tract Infection*.

METHOD

The nine steps when writing outcome standards for a concept unit of care are:

1. Define the unit of care.
2. Specify the time frame.
3. Identify the goals of the nursing care.
4. Identify the positive outcomes expected to occur.
5. Identify the negative outcomes that can be avoided.
6. Specify when you expect each outcome to occur.
7. Clarify the description of the expected outcomes.
8. Combine the outcome standards in a logical order.
9. Establish the validity of the outcome standards.

When you complete the last step, you will have the outcome standards that are ready for implementation.

If you have already developed the process standards for this unit of care, proceed to step 4.

STEP 1
Define the Unit of Care

A carefully defined concept can provide the necessary description to identify the goals of the unit of care. There usually is more than one operational definition of a concept. An **operational definition** of a concept contains a description of the concept in a way that is clear to those nurses developing and implementing the standard.

To test the operational definition of the concept, try to write the goals of the nursing care of the patient. If you have difficulty doing this, you may need to revise the operational definition you have written. For example, an operational definition of a patient who is immobilized is the person who is on bedrest or not actively ambulating. This patient has the potential for a urinary tract infection because of urinary stasis. Others at risk for a urinary tract infection are those who:

1. Are not correctly doing perineal hygiene
2. Have an infection elsewhere in the body
3. Are not drinking enough fluids

Thus, the patient experiencing any one of the predisposing factors or health problems would need the unit of care *Potential for Urinary Tract Infection* on his plan of care.

STEP 2
Specify the Time Frame

Every unit of care requires a time frame. A definite time frame can assist you in identifying the appropriate goals, interventions, and observations of nursing care. As the patient moves along the health-illness-health continuum, the patient's needs for nursing care change. For example, suppose you are developing units of care for the concept *Peri-Operative Care*. You need to develop one unit of care for the preoperative assessment of the patient, the care during surgery, and the immediate postoperative period in the post-anesthesia room as the patient returns to consciousness.

To identify the time frame of the unit of care you are developing, ask yourself:

- At what identifiable time periods will the patient require a different unit of care?
- When must I change the nursing care of this patient as the status of the patient's health changes?

The time frame may already be defined as part of the operational definition of the concept. For the concept *Potential for Urinary Tract Infection*, the time frame is not required, as you would implement this unit of care when a patient has a health problem or is receiving therapy that might result in a urinary tract infection. After you have done this, proceed to step 3.

STEP 3
Identify the Goals of the Nursing Care

The goals assist in further defining the nursing care related to a concept and thus provide a frame of reference for writing outcomes. A **goal** is an explicit statement describing exactly what you plan to accomplish with your nursing care in relation to the patient, patient's family, or patient's environment. As you study the concept and its definition, ask yourself:

- How can nursing care help this patient?

Prevention of complications is a major emphasis of nursing care. The goals for the *Potential for Urinary Tract Infection* are:

- The patient will not experience inflammation of the urinary meatus.
- The patient will not experience a urinary stasis.
- The patient does not have a urinary tract infection.
- The patient is well-hydrated.

Note: The time for achievement of these goals is at all times.

After completing this step, you are ready to develop the outcomes related to these goals.

STEP 4
Identify the Positive Outcomes That Are Expected to Occur

Before beginning to write positive outcomes, you may want to review "Types of Positive Outcomes" and "The Expected Outcomes " in section 1 of this chapter.

To identify positive outcomes, ask yourself:

- What positive outcomes can I expect if this goal is implemented as planned?

Positive outcomes are readily identified when the goals are well-defined. Therefore, if you have trouble answering this question, review the goals to ascertain if they can be specified further.

For each goal of the nursing care related to the concept *Potential for Urinary Tract Infection*, the following question needs to be answered:

- What positive outcomes will occur if the goal is met?

For example, the positive outcomes for the goal *the patient is well hydrated* are:

- The skin and mucous membranes have good turgor.
- The mucous membranes are moist.
- The amount and characteristics of the urine are within normal limits.

(These outcomes are examples of Positive Outcomes Type 2). After you have identified all the positive outcomes for every goal, go on to the next step.

STEP 5
Identify the Negative Outcomes That Can Be Avoided

Before proceeding with this step, you may want to review "Types of Negative Outcomes" in section 1 of this chapter. To identify the negative outcomes that can be prevented if your nursing care plan is implemented, ask yourself:

• What negative outcomes can I avoid if this goal is implemented as planned?

Now identify the negative outcome related to the goal *the patient will not experience an inflammation of the urinary meatus*. The negative outcome is written with the word "not" before the complication *inflammation of the urinary meatus*. (This is an example of Negative Outcome Type 9).

Outcome standards concerning negative outcomes are written so that when they are used for evaluation, the answer "yes" means the patient does *not* have a negative outcome. Two other examples of Negative Outcome Type 9 are:

• The patient does not have urinary stasis.

• The patient does not have a urinary tract infection.

These outcome statements, as the one preceding it, are written in a form for ease in the evaluation of care.

After you have written all the negative outcomes as outcome statements, proceed to step 6.

STEP 6
Specify When You Expect Each Outcome to Occur

You may wish to review "When the Outcome Will Occur" in section 1 of this chapter. Then review each outcome statement and ask yourself:

• When can I expect this outcome to occur?

All the goals in the example concern the maintenance of renal function at pre-immobility function (Positive Outcome Type 2) and the prevention of urinary complications (Negative Outcome Type 9). Because these goals concern the maintenance of the patient's physiological functions at pre-illness levels and prevention of complications, positive outcomes related to these goals should be able to be observed at all times. Thus, if your nursing care is effective, the patient will experience the following outcomes *at all times*:

• The patient is well-hydrated.

• The skin and mucous membranes have good turgor.

• The patient does not have an inflammation of the urinary meatus.

• The patient does not have urinary stasis.

• The patient does not have a urinary tract infection.

In this example, it is not necessary to specify when the outcomes will occur, since they should be present at all times. For most outcome statements you will need to specify the time.

STEP 7
Clarify the Description of the Expected Outcomes

Before beginning this step, you may want to review "How the Outcome Can Be Detected" in section 1 of this chapter. Examine each of the outcome statements and clarify the description of the outcome as needed by the nurses in your agency. Remember, you need to make the outcome statement only as specific as is needed for every nurse who implements the unit of care. The italicized phrases in the following statements specify what needs to be observed to identify whether the outcome standard has been met.

- The patient does not have an inflammation of the urinary meatus, as indicated by an absence of *redness, edema, warmth, and discomfort on the perineal area around the meatus.*
- The patient does not have urinary stasis, as indicated by *urinary output adequate in relation to intake of fluid, at least 30cc/hour.*
- The patient does not have a urinary tract infection, as indicated by absence of:
    a. *Discomfort in the costovertebral area*
    b. *Chills*
    c. *Frequency of urination*
    d. *Urgency of urination*
    e. *Burning on urination*

    Amount and characteristics of the urine are within normal limits.
- The patient is well-hydrated, as indicated by:
    a. *The skin and mucous membranes have good turgor.*
    b. *The mucous membranes are moist.*

Note: For patients who have abnormal responses because of pre-existing pathology, use admission baseline or previous assessment for comparing with outcome data.

The previous statement is a qualifying statement that is needed to make the outcome appropriate for all patients experiencing *Potential for Urinary Tract Infection.* For further explanation of qualifying statements, see chapter 6.

After including the necessary specification for each of the outcome statements, you have written outcome standards. Go on to the next step.

STEP 8
Combine the Outcome Standards in a Logical Order

The completed unit of care includes the title, lists the goals, and combines the outcome standards in a logical order. There are several ways you can organize the outcome standards you have written. You can group those outcomes that are observed together or you can list the outcome standards in the chronological order of their observation. Because the focus of the goals of this unit of care is the maintenance of the patient's health status unaffected by the patient's health problem, you should be able to observe the outcome listed in the standards *at all times*. Thus, the standards are arranged in relation to the source of data needed to confirm that the standard was met.

Unit of Care

Potential for Urinary Tract Infection

Goals

1. The patient will not experience inflammation of the urinary meatus.
2. The patient will not experience a urinary stasis.
3. The patient is well-hydrated.
4. The patient does not have a urinary tract infection.

Note: The time for achievement of these goals is *at all times*.

Outcome Standards

1. The patient does not have an inflammation of the urinary meatus, as indicated by an absence of redness, edema, warmth, and discomfort of the perineal area around the meatus.
2. The patient does not have a urinary tract infection, as indicated by absence of:
   a. Discomfort in the costovertebral area
   b. Chills
   c. Frequency of urination
   d. Urgency of urination
   e. Burning on urination

   The amount and characteristics of the urine are within normal limits.

3. The patient does not have urinary stasis, as indicated by: urinary output adequate in relation to intake of fluid, a minimum of 30cc/hour.

4. The patient is well-hydrated, as indicated by:

    a. The skin and mucous membranes have good turgor.

    b. The mucous membranes are moist.

Note: For patients with abnormal responses because of preexisting pathology, use admission baseline or previous assessment for comparing with outcome data.

After you have combined the outcome standards together in the way thay can best be used, go on to step 9.

STEP 9
Establish the Validity of the Outcome Standards

Although you have developed outcome standards, they are not yet valid. Follow the method described in chapter 5 to establish the validity of the outcome standards you have written.

Now you need to decide whether to proceed to the next section, "Writing Outcome Standards for a Nursing Diagnosis, Health Problem, or Patient Care Need Unit of Care," or to read "Writing Process Standards for a Concept Unit of Care" in chapter 2.

SECTION 5

Writing Outcome Standards for a Nursing Diagnosis, Health Problem, or Patient Care Need Unit of Care

There are several methods used to organize the content of care plans. Many nurses are designing units of care related to the nursing diagnoses, while others construct units of care related to health problems or patient care needs. Some nurses develop units of care of all types. While the labels of the units of care change over time, the interventions and observations you have written for one type of label can be used for another type unless new interventions for the unit of care been identified. When the **Nursing Diagnosis** approach is implemented, the titles of the units of care must be defined for the nurses writing the standards to ensure clarity of understanding. A **nursing diagnosis** can be defined as a clinical judgment about individual, family, or community responses to actual or potential health problems/life processes.[1] Some nurses plan patient care using health problems and patient care needs. A **health problem** or **patient care need** can be defined as a collection of signs and symptoms that, taken together, constitute a picture of ill health or health care required by the patient. The patient care need or problem is expressed in a word or phrase that triggers in the mind of the nurse a picture of the patient care need or problem and the nursing care pertinent to its resolution. An example of titles for a unit of care containing the same interventions and observations related to each type are:

a. Nursing Diagnosis: Sleep Pattern Disturbance[2]

b. Health Problem: Insomnia

c. Patient Care Need: Need for Sleep

As you ponder the approach to be used for the titles of units of care, review the care plans being designed for patients in your agency. If the nurses consistently use patient care needs when planning care, this is the approach to use. Also, review the legal and accrediting requirements for your agency to determine if there are specific requirements for labeling units of care. This information, as well as the nurses' preferences, will assist you in your identification of the labels for the units of care you are writing. The one principle that must be followed is that the nurses implementing the units of care understand the content in the same way as those writing the standards for the unit of care.

Now proceed to study the method for writing outcome standards related to a nursing diagnosis, health problem and patient care need.

METHOD

The nine steps in writing outcome standards for a nursing diagnosis, health problem, or need unit of care are:

1. Define the unit of care.

2. Specify the time frame.

3. Identify the goals of the nursing care.

4. Identify the positive outcomes that are expected to occur.

5. Identify the negative outcomes that can be avoided.

6. Specify when you expect each outcome to occur.

7. Clarify the description of the expected outcomes.
8. Combine the outcome standards in a logical order.
9. Establish the validity of the outcome standards.

When you complete step 9, you will have valid outcome standards that are ready to be implemented. If you have already developed process standards for the nursing care related to this health problem, begin with step 4.

STEP 1
Define the Unit of Care

A definition of the nursing diagnosis, patient care need, or health problem is usually required for clarity of understanding of the unit of care. The definition must be as meaningful to the nurses implementing the standards as those nurses who designed the unit of care. In addition, the unit of care should be defined in such a way that the goals of nursing care can be easily derived from the definition. To illustrate the method of writing standards, the example unit of care can be described as a nursing diagnosis—*Fluid Volume Deficit*.[3] It can also be titled *Dehydration* (health problem) or patient care *Need for Fluid Volume*. Regardless of the title for this unit of care, the operational definition that can be used for writing standards is that the patient is experiencing symptoms from a significant fluid loss from his body.

After you have defined the unit of care, proceed to step 2.

STEP 2
Specify the Time Frame

Every unit of care has a time frame. As the patient progresses along the health-illness-health continuum, the nursing care required by the patient also changes. For example, a patient has one unit of care for the postoperative care from postanesthesia until ambulation and another unit of care from ambulation until discharge, because the needs of the patients change as the patient progresses after surgery. On the other hand, for some units of care the time frame can be omitted because there is only one time frame for this problem or need. The unit of care for Insomnia, or Need for Sleep, does not require a time frame. The interventions for this unit of care are operational when this unit of care is added to the patient's care plan. If the time frame for the unit of care you are developing has not been specified, do it now. Ask yourself:

- At what identifiable time periods will the patient require a different unit of care?

- When must I change the nursing care of this patient as the status of the patient's health changes?

For example, the time frame for the unit of care for a patient with the following is when the patient is experiencing this unit of care.

- Nursing Diagnosis: Fluid Volume Loss
- Health Problem: Dehydration
- Patient Care Need: Need for Fluid Volume
- After you have identified the time frame for the unit of care you are designing, proceed to step 3.

STEP 3
Identify the Goals of the Nursing Care

The goals further define the nursing care of a patient experiencing a unit of care and thus provide guidelines for the identification of outcomes. A **goal** is an explicit statement describing exactly what you plan to accomplish with your nursing care. As you think about a nursing diagnosis, health problem, or patient care need and its definition, ask yourself:

- How can nursing care help a patient having this?
  - Nursing Diagnosis: Fluid Volume Loss
  - Health Problem: Dehydration
  - Patient Care Need: Need for Fluid Volume

The patient who has experienced a loss of fluid volume will require the following goals:

- The patient's level of hydration will improve.
- The patient will be comfortable.
- The patient's family will be kept informed of the patient's status.
- Before discharge, the patient will be able to describe how to prevent a decreased level of hydration.
- The patient will not experience fluid overload.

Note: When the goals are individualized for a specific patient, the exact date for the achievement of the goal must be defined.

STEP 4
Identify the Positive Outcomes
That Are Expected to Occur

You may wish to reread "Types of Positive Outcomes" and "The Expected Outcome" in section 1 of this chapter before proceeding with this step. To identify the positive outcomes of the nursing care for this patient, ask yourself:

- What positive outcomes can I expect if this goal is implemented as planned?

Positive outcomes are easily identified if the goals of the unit of care are well-defined. Thus, if you have difficulty answering this question, review the goals you have written and revise them as needed. Now identify the outcomes related to each goal.

Consider this goal: *The patient's level of hydration will improve.* Ask yourself:

- What positive outcomes can I expect if this goal is implemented as planned?

The positive outcomes related to this goal are:

- The patient's level of hydration is improving.
- The patient's lab results are within normal limits.
- The patient's urinary output is 30cc per hour.

(These outcomes are examples of the type of Positive Outcome Type 1, *an improvement in the health status of the patient* and Type 2, *maintenance of the patient's health status unaffected by the patient's health problem* (see section 1 of this chapter).

The goal *the patient will be comfortable* has the following positive outcomes:

- The patient's needs for comfort are being met.
- The patient states, when asked, that his needs are being met.

(These outcomes are examples of the type of Positive Outcome Type 3, *an increase in the patient's psychological and physiological comfort.*)

The goal *the patient's family will be kept informed of the patient's status*, if met, will result in this outcome:

- The patient's family when asked, state they are informed concerning the patient's status.

(This is an example of the type of Positive Outcome Type 11, *an increase in the family's psychological and physiological comfort.*)

The outcome for the goal *the patient will be able to describe how to prevent a decreased level of hydration* is:

- The patient and family can describe how to prevent loss of fluid volume.

(This is an example of the type of Positive Outcome Type 4, *an increase in the patient's knowledge of the patient and/or family needed to prevent a health problem.*)

After you have identified all the positive outcomes for every goal, review all the goals and outcomes together to ascertain whether you have identified all the outcomes. Then proceed to the next step.

STEP 5
Identify the Negative Outcomes
That Can Be Avoided

Before proceeding, you may wish to review "Types of Negative Outcomes" in section 1 of this chapter. To identify the negative outcomes preventable with excellent nursing care, ask yourself:

- What negative outcomes can be avoided if the nursing care related to this goal are implemented as planned?

The negative outcome that can be prevented as defined by the goal *the patient will not experience fluid overload* is:

- *The patient is not experiencing fluid overload.* Or, the outcome can be written as *absence of fluid overload.*

(This is an example of the type of prevention of Negative Outcome Type 9, *complications.*) All negative outcomes are written so that a "yes" response to the standard means the patient experienced a positive outcome. This is done to ensure clarity during the evaluation of the care related to the outcome.

After you have written all the negative outcomes, go on to step 6.

STEP 6
Specify When You Expect
Each Outcome to Occur

Before proceeding with this step, you may wish to review "When the Outcome Will Occur" in section 1 of this chapter. Now review each of the following outcomes and ask yourself:

- When can I expect this outcome to occur?

Because the following outcomes relate to improvement in the patient's health status, provision of comfort for the patient/family and prevention of complications, the "when" is *at all times*.

- The patient's level of hydration is improving.
- The patient's lab results are within normal limits.
- The patient's urinary output is 30cc per hour.

Note: *If not, the physician has been notified.*

- The patient is not experiencing fluid overload: increasing weight, elevated blood pressure, peripheral edema, dyspnea, cough, pulmonary edema, nausea, or vomiting. *If any of these signs and symptoms are present, the physician has been notified.* (This action statement is included so the clinicians remember to notify the physician when significant changes occur in the patient's condition.)
- The patient's needs for comfort are being met.
- The patient's family says it is informed of the patient's status and changes in the patient's condition.

When the phrase "at all times" is attached to an outcome, the positive outcome should be present at any time you visit the patient.

The outcome *the patient and family can describe how to prevent a decreased level of hydration* must be achieved before discharge. The patient and family are interviewed several days before discharge to identify their knowledge level concerning this outcome. If they are unsure what to do after discharge, there is time to reteach them or write a referral before the patient is discharged.

Note: When the outcomes are individualized for a specific patient, the exact date for the achievement of the outcome must be defined.

When you have completed this step, proceed to step 7.

STEP 7
Clarify the Description of the Expected Outcomes

As you may remember, each outcome statement should be written as specifically as needed by every staff member implementing the care. The following outcomes contain the necessary specification that might need to be included for staff to evaluate the care given using these outcomes:

- The patient's level of hydration is improving. If not, the physician has been notified. Observations related to the patient's level of hydration are:
  a. Skin turgor
  b. Dry skin and mucous membranes
  c. Specific gravity of the urine
  d. Quality and rate of the pulse

Compare the observations made with the last time the patient's level of hydration was evaluated. A comparison with a prior assessment is necessary to identify whether the patient's fluid volume is returning to normal.

- The patient's lab results are within normal limits. If not, the physician has been notified. If a lab result is abnormal, compare it to a previous result and the results of the patient's lab test on admission. The result is the same or improved since the last test.

- The patient's urinary output is 30cc per hour; if not, the physician has been notified. Compare the observations made with the last time the patient's urinary output was evaluated. The result is the same or improved since last observation.

- The patient's needs for comfort are being met if:
  a. There is an absence of dry skin, lip irritation, and mucous membranes of the mouth.
  b. The patient says, when asked, that his needs are being met.
  c. The temperature of the room is comfortable for the patient.
  d. The patient says, when asked, that he is receiving assistance with activities of daily living as needed.

- When asked, the patient's family says it is informed of the patient's status and changes in the patient's condition.

- The patient's family has expressed no complaints regarding a lack of information concerning the patient's progress.

- Before discharge, the patient and family can describe how to prevent a decreased level of hydration:
  a. Amount of fluid intake per day required
  b. Method(s) of meeting the fluid goal
  c. Observations to be reported to the physician (causes of loss of fluid)

    d. Family assistance required or referral to community agency

- The patient is not experiencing fluid overload: rapid weight gain, shortness of breath, or increased blood pressure. If any of these symptoms are present, the physician has been notified.

You will note that some of these outcomes contain the phrase "the physician has been notified." This phrase is a qualifying statement that defines the responsibility of the health professional who can intervene if the outcome is becoming negative. It is important to identify what health discipline should intervene if outcomes are becoming negative, so there is no time lost in intervention. For more information on qualifying statements read chapter 6, section 1.

STEP 8
Combine the Outcome Standards
in a Logical Order

The completed unit of care includes the title, lists its goals, and combines the outcome standards in a logical order. There are several ways to organize outcome standards. You can list the standards in the chronological order of their observation or you can group those outcomes together that are observed together. You need to list the standards in an order that is most helpful to the nurses implementing them. These outcome standards are listed in relation to the source of data for each outcome.

Unit of Care

- Nursing diagnosis: Fluid Volume Deficit
- Health problem: Dehydration
- Patient care need: Need for Fluid Volume

Goals

1. The patient's level of hydration will improve.
2. The patient will be comfortable.
3. The patient's family will be kept informed of the patient's status.
4. Before discharge, the patient will be able to describe how to prevent a decreased level of hydration.
5. The patient will not experience fluid overload.

Note: When the goals are individualized for a specific patient, the exact date for the achievement of the goal must be defined.

Outcome Standards

- At all times the patient's level of hydration is improving. If not, the physician has been notified. Observations related to the patient's level of hydration are:
  a. Skin turgor
  b. Dry skin and mucous membranes
  c. Specific gravity of the urine
  d. Quality and rate of the pulse

(Compare the observations made with the last time the patient's level of hydration was evaluated.)

- The patient is not experiencing fluid overload: rapid weight gain, shortness of breath, or increased blood pressure. If any of these symptoms are present, the physician has been notified.

- The patient's lab results are within normal limits. If not, the physician has been notified. (If a lab result is abnormal, compare it to a previous result and the results of the patient's lab test on admission. The result is the same or improved since the last test.)

- The patient's urinary output is 30cc per hour; if not, the physician has been notified. (Compare the observations made with the last time the patient's urinary output was evaluated. The result is the same or improved since last observation.)

- The patient's needs for comfort are being met:
  a. There is an absence of dry skin, lip irritation, and mucous membranes of the mouth.
  b. The patient says, when asked, that his needs are being met.
  c. The temperature of the room is comfortable for the patient.
  d. The patient says, when asked, that he is receiving assistance with activities of daily living as needed.

- When asked, the patient's family says it is informed of the patient's status and changes in the patient's condition.

- The patient's family has expressed no complaints regarding a lack of information concerning the patient's progress.

- Before discharge, the patient and family can describe:
  a. How to prevent a decreased level of hydration
  b. Amount of fluid intake per day required
  c. Method(s) of meeting the fluid goal

    d. Observations to be reported to the physician (causes of loss of fluid)

    e. Family assistance required or referral to community agency

Note: When the outcomes are individualized for a specific patient, the exact date for the achievement of the outcome must be defined.

STEP 9
Establish the Validity of the Outcome Standards

Although you have developed outcome standards, they are not valid. Read chapter 5 to establish the validity of these outcomes.

    You have completed the section on how to write outcome standards for a nursing diagnosis, health problem, or patient care need unit of care. Now you need to decide whether to read "Writing Process Standards for a Nursing Diagnosis, Health Problem, or Patient Care Need Unit of Care" in chapter 2 or another chapter in the book.

NOTES

1. Carpenito, Lynda Juall. *Nursing diagnosis: Application to clinical practice* (4th ed.), p.6. New York: J.B. Lipincott and Co., 1992.

2. Ibid., p.776.

3. Ibid., p.379.

4

Writing Standards for Interdisciplinary Units of Care

Optimal health care occurs when all health professionals contribute the care related to their discipline in the correct sequence that results in positive outcomes for a patient and her family. To address all the health problems of the patient, it is essential that all members of the health team:

- Possess the knowledge and skills needed to provide care related to all the patient's health problems
- Refer the patient to health professionals when the patient needs interventions not available at this health agency
- Assume responsibility for:
  - a. Assessment of the patient
  - b. Implementation of the standards of their discipline
  - c. Evaluation/reassessment of the patient's status

The optimum in health care doesn't always happen. For example, a patient was admitted to the hospital for a mitral valve repair. The first 36 hours were uneventful for the patient. Then he was transferred from the Surgical Intensive Care Unit to a Medical Intensive Care Unit to begin active participation in his recuperation. The cardiac rehabilitation team and the cardiac surgical team gave the patient and his family different answers to questions related to the patient's diet, activity, and other aspects of his care after discharge. The family received confusing and contradictory answers when they asked health team members about his progress and the care being implemented, especially when the patient was not making satisfactory progress. For example, the patient experienced pulmonary edema when he was in the stepdown unit. He was moved back to the Medical Intensive Care Unit. The nurses and physicians did not have an accurate picture of the patient's fluid balance and hemodynamic parameters 6 hours after the patient was transferred. And when the internist diagnosed that the patient was experiencing an untoward reaction to one of his medications, the surgical team responsible for the patient's plan of care did not read the physician's recommended orders or change his medications for more than 48 hours after the orders had been written.

Throughout his postoperative stay, the patient had difficulty swallowing because of the trauma from the endotracheal tube and did not receive adequate nutrition. Although the cardiac surgical team and cardiac rehabilitation team were aware of this problem, nothing was done. This problem was not mentioned on the referral to the community health agency on his discharge. Therefore, the problem worsened in the two weeks following his discharge, causing the patient to be readmitted to the hospital.

The leader of the health team was not consistently available to coordinate the patient's plan of care even if the clinicians had developed an interdisciplinary plan of care for this patient. The health team did not confer on its assessments, implementation, and evaluations. Thus, the talents of individual health team members were not used to design and implement an effective plan for the patient's care.

In summary, there are some major issues that need to be resolved to achieve a fully effective health team.

SECTION 1

Issues Related to
Writing Interdisciplinary Standards

WHO IS THE LEADER/ARBITER OF THE TEAM?

To ensure that the patient's care is implemented effectively and in a timely fashion, every patient needs a health professional to coordinate the work of the other team members. This clinician becomes the arbiter when there are contradictory approaches recommended by members of the team.

In many situations the health professional that spends the least time at the facility is the leader of the health team. This form of coordination leads to overlaps and gaps in services for patients. It is vital that the leader of the team for a patient's plan of care must be actively involved with the implementation of the patient's care.

WHO DOES THE ASSESSMENT OF THE PATIENT?

Every health professional has certain knowledge/skills that define his or her health discipline. Some of these are shared by other health professionals, while others are distinctly different. It is essential that the team decide who is going to do which assessments to avoid gaps and redundancies in the assessments.

As clinicians' roles evolve, their functions change. They might no longer do certain assessments or might have new assessment duties that overlap with those done by others. Therefore, it cannot be assumed that all aspects of the patient's health status are being assessed.

Unless the team members discuss changes in their roles when they occur, there will be gaps or redundancies in the assessment of the patient, which can lead to a plan of care that does not meet all the patient's health needs. Communication is essential to keep the assessment valid and useful in interdisciplinary planning.

DO MEMBERS OF THE HEALTH TEAM ASSUME RESPONSIBILITY FOR ASSESSMENT, IMPLEMENTATION, AND EVALUATION RELATED TO THEIR DISCIPLINE?

A clinician represents her discipline and brings the knowledge of this health discipline to the assessment of the patient and the planning, implementation, and the evaluation of the patient's care. Those clinicians implementing the plan of care may not have the same level and type of expertise as the clinicians designing the plan. When this occurs, the patient does not receive the full benefit of the knowledge and skills of each health discipline that would make the care more effective.

Thus, for most health problems and needs of a patient, a clinician from each health discipline should be involved in all aspects of the patient's care. Even if a health discipline does not need to contribute interventions to the plan of care, one of its clinicians should contribute to the assessment and the design of the plan.

A major block to interdisciplinary planning in many health teams is the belief of certain health professionals that they know what interventions should be done by other members of the health team, an obvious source of controversy. These health professionals believe they should participate only in the design of the plan of care while others on the team should do the assessment, implementation, and evaluation of outcomes.

To avoid controversy, a guiding principle for a health team is that each discipline is responsible for planning, implementing, and evaluating the care their clinicians can provide for the patient. **One discipline cannot decide what interventions will be implemented by another discipline**. The leader of a health team may need to set additional guidelines for group functioning to keep the team focused when writing the standards or during interdisciplinary planning.

WHAT LABELS WILL BE GIVEN TO THE UNITS OF CARE?

Health professionals have various ways for titling health problems and patient care needs. A common approach to titling units of care relates to the *medical model* because of the historical approach of using the *medical diagnosis* for labeling all aspects of the patient's plan of care. *Nursing diagnosis* is a method for titling units of care that is recognized by nurses but may not be accepted by other health team members. Accrediting agencies may define how the units of care should be titled.

Another consideration when titling a unit of care is the time frame, which might vary from one discipline to another. For some disciplines a unit of care may last from admission to discharge because the interventions implemented by this discipline remain the same during this time period.

Other disciplines have designed interventions related to more specific problems with a shorter time frame. For example, physicians and psychologists can create a unit of care for *Depression* that lasts from admission to discharge. Nursing, on the other hand, may have these nursing diagnoses that could be selected for a *Patient with Depression:*

1. Sleep Pattern Disturbances

2. Potential for Violence
3. Sleep Pattern Disturbance
4. Altered Thought Processes
5. Impaired Social Interaction
6. Hopelessness
7. Knowledge Deficit R/T Medications

A social worker might have the following units of care for this same patient:

1. Depression, Hopelessness or Low Self-Esteem
2. Patient Needs Financial Resources
3. Problematic Family Relationships
4. Need for Service or Item
5. Inadequate Family Involvement/Support

An occupational therapist might have the following units of care for this patient:

1. Budgeting
2. Group Interaction: Tactile Stimulation
3. Activities of Daily Living: Personal Care
4. Recreational Group: Community Facilities

In this example you will note that there are some health problems/patient care needs that are interdisciplinary. For other health problems/patient care needs, one discipline *alone* may address the patient's need or problem.

IS THE AMOUNT OF TIME CONTRIBUTED BY EACH OF THE HEALTH TEAM MEMBERS CONSISTENT WITH THE AMOUNT OF TIME *REQUIRED* TO PROVIDE QUALITY CARE FOR THE PATIENT?

In some facilities, due to financial constraints, there is only a skeleton of a health team. When this occurs, there are gaps in all phases of patient care. The team needs to identify these gaps and identify ways to eliminate them.

When the standards for all aspects of interdisciplinary health care are defined in a facility, the number and level of clinicians required from each health discipline to implement these standards will have been defined.

After the standards have been written, budgets may need to be modified to ensure that the patient can have a complete assessment from all of the health team members that can be planned, implemented, and evaluated. (See "Interdisciplinary Planning" in chapter 7.)

SECTION 2
Writing Content Standards for Assessment

The first step in interdisciplinary planning is the assessment of the patient by all members of the health team. While the assessments may be done at various time periods after the patient is admitted to the health agency, all health professionals must assess the patient prior to developing the patient's plan of care. If there is a change in the patient's health status, all health team members need to assess the patient's present status to ensure the interventions on the new plan reflect the patient's current needs/problems.

To prevent unnecessary duplication in the data collected, the health team members need to define for each of the units of care which data items will be obtained from the patient by each health discipline. While the subjective data items may require more than one health professional's assessment, there are many objective data items that are often collected by several health professionals. This redundancy decreases the efficiency of the health team. It also causes unnecessary fatigue for patients by repeatedly asking them for the same information.

After each discipline has identified its list of data to be collected, content standards are developed for all data collection tools to provide consistency from one clinician to another. The content standards define the categories of data essential to the provision of care.

The assessment categories must be related to the patient's health status for each unit of care. If an assessment category concerning a unit of care is missing, the health professional may not select this unit of care when it is indicated for a patient. Thus, after you have finished writing standards for all units of care, review the assessment tools you have developed in relation to:

    a. The selection of units of care during care planning

    b. The patient outcomes of all units of care for reassessment and evaluation after the patient has received care

There are two major types of data collection: *focused assessment* and *total assessment*. A **focused assessment** is the data collection related to one health problem or patient care need. A **total assessment** is data collection concerning all characteristics of the patient and factors external to the patient that should be considered when planning and implementing care. This is necessary to identify the patient's initial needs/health problems and to establish the baseline that will be used to identify the patient's progress after she has received care. Because assessment data are a baseline for the next assessment and will be used to identify the patient's response to therapy and progress toward the patient outcomes, the categories of data in the assessment should include all the outcomes listed in the outcome standards.

At periodic intervals the health professional can use a focused assessment to collect data about the patient's status and match it with the baseline to identify whether the patient has experienced improvement in one or more dimensions of her health status. At these periodic assessments the health professional should determine whether the patient's plan of care is meeting her needs or should be modified if she is not making satisfactory progress.

A *Patient with Chronic Pain* is the example unit of care that will illustrate the method. Because chronic pain has a negative effect on many of the patient's functions and lifestyle over a long period of time, a total assessment should be done for the initial assessment of the patient having chronic pain. A focused assessment can be done at subsequent periodic intervals to identify whether the patient is progressing. When there is a significant change in the patient's health status another total assessment should be done.

METHOD

The method of writing content standards related to obtaining data from patients consists of four steps:

1. Define the patient's health situation.
2. Identify the goals of data collection.
3. Identify the items of data collection.
4. Assign responsibility for data collection.
5. Combine the content standards in a logical order.
6. Establish the validity of standards.

After you have completed step 4, the standards you have written will be ready for implementation. Now begin with step 1.

STEP 1
Define the Patient's Health Situation

An accurate description of the patient's health situation can help you identify the goals of data collection. This description should be brief but must
contain the details necessary to provide a picture of the patient. Included in
the patient's health situation is a description of the philosophy of the health
agency and the setting in which the care will be implemented. Thus, the
assessment tool for the patient having chronic pain who is immobilized in a
long-term care agency will contain *some* but not all of the items on the tool
used to assess the patient who is ambulatory and receiving care at an outpatient clinic.

After you have specified the patient's health situation, go on to step 2.

STEP 2
Identify the Goals of Data Collection

A major consideration in relation to the goals of data collection are the types
of health services that can be provided for patients by this agency. The goals
of the services may be maintenance of the patient's health or the treatment
of acutely and chronically ill. Because the therapy for maintaining the patient's health status is different from treatment of an acutely ill patient, some
of the data collected from patients are different. It is important that patients
are not asked for information that is non-essential for the provision of
services.

You also may want to review the definition of a goal. A **goal** is an explicit
statement describing what data you want to obtain from the patient. Thus,
the type of data you collect from a patient will include the nature of the
patient's health situation, whether you need a focused or total assessment,
and the goals for data collection.

To identify the goals, you need to answer these questions:

- What do I need to know about this patient
    a. To develop her plan of care?
    b. To teach her what she needs to know to control her pain?
    c. To assist her to maintain or modify her present lifestyle?
    d. To assist the family to be supportive?

The goals for the *Patient in Chronic Pain* are:

- The patient will be able to control her pain.

- The patient will be able to identify the factors/situations/persons that increase, precipitate, or decrease her pain.
- The patient will be able to pursue or modify her lifestyle before pain began to meet her present needs.
- The family will receive the assistance to support the patient.
- The patient and/or family will understand how to implement the patient's plan of care.
- The patient will not experience preventable side effects of therapy or complications.
- The family will be assisted in modifying their lifestyle (see p. 87) as needed.

Now proceed to step 3.

STEP 3
Identify the Items of Data Collection

You are ready to identify the items of data to be collected. As you examine each goal, ask yourself:

- What data must I collect to meet this goal?
- What data are essential to obtain from the patient and family related to the patient experiencing chronic pain?

When you have obtained answers to these questions, you will have identified the content standards for this data collection tool.

The following items should be included in an interdisciplinary assessment of a *Patient with Chronic Pain*.

- General history and physical examination related to the
    a. Causes of the pain
    b. Effect of the pain on the patient's ability to function
- Family's lifestyle before patient experienced pain
    a. Work of family members
    b. Leisure of family members
    c. Each member's ability to meet family responsibilities
    d. Relationships
    e. Responses to the patient's pain
    f. Cultural beliefs about pain
    g. Religious beliefs about pain

- Patient's perception of pain
  - a. Onset
  - b. Duration
  - c. Intensity–use pain scale
  - d. Location
  - e. Signs and symptoms
  - f. Ability to be distracted
  - g. Prior experiences with pain
- Factors/situations that increase pain
- Factors/situations that decrease pain
- Patient's level of mobility prior to experiencing pain
- Patient's level of mobility now
- Patient's ability to do Activities of Daily Living prior to experiencing pain
- Patient's ability to do Activities of Daily Living now
- Patient's lifestyle *prior to pain*
  - a. Ability to work
  - b. Ability to meet family responsibilities
  - c. Leisure activities
  - d. Perception of:
    1. Family support
    2. Each family member's responses to her pain
  - e. Sleep patterns
  - f. Nutrition
  - g. Elimination
- Patient's lifestyle *now*
  - a. Ability to work
  - b. Ability to meet family responsibilities
  - c. Leisure activities
  - d. Perception of
    1. Family support
    2. Each family member's responses to her pain
  - e. Sleep patterns
  - f. Nutrition
  - g. Elimination

- Patient's responses to
  a. Use of art therapy
  b. Use of music therapy
  c. Stress management techniques
  d. Use of massage
  e. Use of heat and cold
  f. Use of special breathing patterns
  g. Guided imagery
  h. Biofeedback
  i. Use of resources
  j. Hypnosis
  k. Relaxation response

After the data items have been identified, go on to step 4.

STEP 4
Assign Responsibility for Data Collection

Each discipline needs to develop data collection tools containing the items for which it is responsible. Then proceed to the next step.

STEP 5
Combine the Content Standards in a Logical Order

The completed unit of care identifies the patient's health situation, lists the goals of the communication, and combines the content standards in a logical order by health discipline. Review all the items of data collection for completeness and list them in an order for interdisciplinary assessment. The following order is just one way the standards can be listed.

Patient's Health Problem

Chronic Pain

Goals

1. The patient will be able to control her pain.
2. The patient will be able to identify the factors/situations that increase and decrease pain.

3. The patient will be able to pursue or modify her previous lifestyle to meet her present needs.
4. The family will receive assistance to support the patient.
5. The patient and/or family will understand how to implement the patient's plan of care.
6. The patient will not experience side effects of therapy or complications.
7. The family will be assisted in modifying its lifestyle as needed.

Content Standards

1. General history and physical examination related to:
   a. Causes of pain
   b. Effect of pain on the patient's ability to function
2. Family's lifestyle *before* patient experienced pain
   a. Work of family members
   b. Leisure of family members
   c. Each member's ability to meet family responsibilities
   d. Relationships
   e. Responses to the patient's pain
   f. Cultural beliefs about pain
   g. Religious beliefs about pain
3. Patient's perception of pain
   a. Onset
   b. Duration
   c. Intensity–use pain scale
   d. Location
   e. Signs and symptoms
   f. Ability to be distracted
   g. Prior experiences with pain
4. Factors/situations that increase pain
5. Factors/situations that decrease pain
6. Patient's level of mobility prior to experiencing pain
7. Patient's level of mobility now
8. Patient's ability to do Activities of Daily Living prior to experiencing pain

9. Patient's ability to do Activities of Daily Living now
10. Patient's lifestyle *prior* to pain
    a. Ability to work
    b. Ability to meet family responsibilities
    c. Leisure activities
    d. Perception of
       1. Family support
       2. Each family member's responses to her pain
    e. Sleep patterns
    f. Nutrition
    g. Elimination
11. Patient's lifestyle *now*
    a. Ability to work
    b. Ability to meet family responsibilities
    c. Leisure activities
    d. Perception of
       1. Family support
       2. Each family member's responses to her pain
    e. Sleep patterns
    f. Nutrition
    g. Elimination
12. Patient's responses to:
    a. Use of art therapy
    b. Use of music therapy
    c. Stress management techniques
    d. Use of massage
    e. Use of heat and cold
    f. Use of special breathing patterns
    g. Guided imagery
    h. Biofeedback
    i. Use of resources
    j. Hypnosis
    k. Relaxation response

STEP 6
Establish the Validity of the Standards

Although you have developed content standards, these standards are not valid. The standards need to be reviewed by three people knowledgeable about the data that must be collected. This step is done to ensure the content validity of the standards. After there is agreement among the experts that these are the content standards, the standards are ready for implementation. You have completed this section.

SECTION 3
Writing Process Standards for Interdisciplinary Units of Care

The **process standards** of interdisciplinary units of care are the interventions and observations that need to be implemented by clinicians of each health discipline related to the goals of the unit of care. Before health team members begin to design interdisciplinary units of care, the clinicians of each health discipline should identify all the interventions and observations implemented for each health problem/patient care need experienced by patients in their agency. If this thinking is done prior to the meeting of the entire health team, the time required for writing the standards should be decreased.

When the team meets, the long- and short-term goals for the units of care can be more easily identified for each unit of care. Then the health team members can discuss the interventions and observations from each discipline for the patient's plan of care.

Interdisciplinary units of care can have various titles for the same problem or need because each health discipline views the unit of care from a different perspective. The team has to agree on a title for each unit of care shared across disciplines. The most common approach is to use health problem/patient care need to define the units of care.

A **health problem/patient care need** can be defined as a collection of signs and symptoms that, taken together, constitute a picture of ill health or health care required by the patient. The patient care need/problem is expressed in a word or phrase that triggers in the mind of the staff a picture of the patient care need/problem and the care pertinent to its resolution. Examples include: *Dehydration/Need for Hydration; Chronic Pain/Need for Pain Relief*; and *Constipation/Need for Increased Gastro-Intestinal Motility*.

METHOD

The ten steps in writing process standards for an interdisciplinary unit of care are:

1. Define the unit of care.
2. Specify the time frame.
3. Identify the goals of care.
4. List the interventions that will meet the goals.
5. Identify the observations related to the patient's responses and the patient's progress.
6. Specify when each intervention and observation needs to be done.
7. Combine the process standards in a logical order.
8. Eliminate suggestions and rationale from the process standards you have written.
9. Identify which health discipline will be responsible for implementing each intervention and observation.
10. Establish the validity of the process standards.

STEP 1
Define the Unit of Care

Selecting a label or title of the health problem/patient care need is the first step in the method. The title of the unit of care must be clear enough that the clinicians from every health discipline implementing the standards will have the same mental picture of the unit of care as those clinicians writing the standards. To test the title, try to write the goals of the care for the patient. If you are unable to define the goals, change the title.

As you decide what titles should be used, review the titles of the units of care on the plans of care being designed for patients in your agency. Also, review the legal and accrediting requirements to determine whether there are specific requirements for the titles of units of care. For example, if reimbursement agencies will provide additional reimbursement for the agency when you use certain titles for the patients' health problems, use these titles to develop your standards.

The unit of care that will be used to demonstrate the method for writing interdisciplinary process standards is *Patient Who Is Experiencing Chronic Pain. Chronic Pain* can be defined as the discomfort experienced by a person over a period of time such that the end to the pain cannot be identified. *Chronic Pain* is further defined by the patient's health status identified during the initial assessment. The pain is severe enough that it affects the patient's health status in bodily areas not affected by the pain and negatively affects the patient's lifestyle and relationships with other people.

After you have selected a title for the unit of care, proceed to step 2.

STEP 2
Specify the Time Frame

Some units of care must have a defined time frame. To identify whether a time frame is needed for this unit of care, ask yourself:

- At what identifiable time periods will the patient require a different unit of care?
- When must I change the care as the patient's health status changes?

In our example, the time frame for the unit of care *Chronic Pain* is defined in the title. The time frame is when the patient is experiencing pain over an extended time period. The pain is not being controlled by the patient and is impairing the quality of her lifestyle and her ability to function. The patient's responses to the chronic pain may also be negatively affecting her family's lifestyle. Further specification of a time frame for this unit of care could be when the patient:

    a. Is terminally ill on bedrest

    b. Has chronic low back pain and is ambulatory

After you have considered a time frame for this unit of care, proceed to step 3.

STEP 3
Identify the Goals of Care

After the time frame of the health problem/patient care need has been defined, the goals of care can be specified. Goals enable you to identify pertinent interventions for the unit of care. A **goal** is an explicit statement describing exactly what you plan to accomplish with the care. To identify the goals related to a health problem/patient care need, think about the care that is appropriate for a patient with chronic pain. Ask yourself:

- What care is appropriate for a patient experiencing chronic pain?
- What care/teaching is needed to assist the patient in maintaining or modifying her lifestyle?

- What care/teaching is needed to assist the patient's family to be supportive to her?

The goals for the patient having *Chronic Pain* are:

- The patient will be able to control her pain.
- The patient will be able to identify the factors/situations/persons that increase, precipitate, or decrease her pain.
- The patient will be able to pursue or modify her prior lifestyle before the pain began to meet her present needs.
- The patient will not experience preventable side effects of therapy or complications.
- The family will receive assistance to support the patient.
- The patient and/or family will understand how to implement the patient's plan of care.
- The family will be assisted in modifying its lifestyle as needed.

Note: When the goals are individualized for a specific patient, the exact date for the achievement of the goal must be defined.

After you have identified the goals, proceed to Step 4.

STEP 4
List the Interventions That Will Meet the Goals

Now that you have identified the goals for the unit of care, identify the interventions that are related to each goal. As you write the interventions, think about the philosophy and overall goals of your health agency.

The philosophy and goals of the health agency as defined by the members of the health team will affect the process standards related to the care of the patient who has chronic pain. For example, while a goal of all health agencies is to reduce or eliminate the chronic pain, the interventions to do so and associated goals will vary from agency to agency. One agency might use acupuncture and humor as interventions, while another agency philosophically would not. Not all the interventions in the example would be implemented for one patient. The most common interventions are listed so that clinicians from various disciplines can select those appropriate to a specific patient.

For each goal, ask yourself:

- What interventions must be implemented to meet this goal?

Let's study the first goal: *The patient will be able to control her pain.*

- What can the health team do to assist the patient to control her pain?

The following interventions are examples of answers to that question:

- Explore interventions used by the patient in the past and her evaluation of their effectiveness.
- Identify the patient's perception of Pain Control.
- Explore the interventions used by the patient in the past and her evaluation of their effectiveness.
- Assist the patient to implement interventions that reduce pain and that are congruent with the patient's cultural and religious beliefs. Some specific interventions to decrease pain are:
  a. Patient-controlled analgesia
  b. Analgesics
  c. Biofeedback
  d. Transcutaneous electric nerve stimulation
  e. Therapeutic touch
  f. Therapeutic massage
  g. Immobilization
  h. Acupuncture
  i. Increasing physical comfort:
    1. Position
    2. Reposition
    3. Exercise to increase and restore function
    4. Time and adjust activities and treatments to allow for optimum comfort
    5. Schedule activities to allow for adequate rest and sleep without interference with pain control schedule

Increased anxiety can heighten perception of pain. Thus, it is essential to assist the patient to implement interventions that decrease anxiety and increase relaxation:
  a. Distraction
  b. Relaxation exercises
  c. Guided imagery
  d. Visualization
  e. Hypnosis
  f. Music therapy

    g. Art therapy

    h. Humor in literature/movies/television

The following are examples of interventions that also help to decrease fear and anxiety:

    a. Encourage the patient to verbalize fears and ask questions about her plan of care.

    b. Explain all procedures/interventions and her participation in them.

    c. Provide the patient with the information that encourages her decisionmaking (when possible) in selecting goals/interventions/activities.

    d. Modify her environment to promote rest and relaxation.

    e. Demonstrate breathing patterns that increase comfort.

    f. Demonstrate stress reduction activities.

- Assist the patient with her activities.
- Time and adjust activities to allow for optimal pain relief.
- Schedule/modify activities to allow for adequate rest and sleep without interference with pain control schedule.

Note: If the patient is on bedrest, the unit of care *Immobilization* will also be required for this patient.

Let's study the second goal: *The patient will be able to identify* the factors/situations/persons that increase, precipitate, or decrease pain. Ask yourself:

- How can the health team assist the patient identify the factors that increase and decrease pain?

These interventions are some of the possible answers to that question:

- Ask the patient to identify the situations, factors, or persons in her environment that increase, precipitate, or decrease her pain.
- Assist the patient to modify or eliminate those situations, factors, or persons that increase or precipitate her pain. Some examples of those interventions are:

    a. Positions that increase comfort

    b. Activities that can be done without increasing pain

    c. Transfer techniques and body mechanics that decrease or eliminate pain

    d. Massage, stroking, or gentle touch that modifies pain conduction

    e. Limited visiting time of persons who increase the patient's stress and anxiety

- Teach the patient how to modify or eliminate those activities, factors, or persons in her environment that increase or precipitate pain.

Then, review the third goal: *The patient will be able to pursue or modify her prior lifestyle before the pain began to meet her present needs.* The interventions are:

- Interview the patient regarding her lifestyle prior to her pain.
- Assist the patient to compare her lifestyle prior to her pain with her present ability to function and identify the modifications, if any, that need to be made to meet her present needs.
- Assist the patient to express her feelings.
- Teach problem solving in relation to modifying her lifestyle prior to pain to meet current needs, when necessary.
- Teach the patient how to set realistic goals.
  - a. Activities of daily living
  - b. Level of mobility
  - c. Possible job modifications
  - d. Financial needs
  - e. Relationships with family
- Assist the patient to identify resources and supportive persons.
- Encourage use of a support system—e.g., family, spiritual adviser.
- Counsel as needed.
- Provide positive reinforcement for achievements.
- Identify the patient's needs for assistive devices.

Now, examine the fourth goal: *The patient will not experience preventable side effects of therapy or complications.* The intervention is:

- Teach the patient and her family the side effects of therapy and the observations that should be reported to the health team (also pertinent to Goal 5).

The following interventions are related to the fifth goal: *The family will receive the assistance needed to support the patient.*

- Listen to each family member's perception of the patient's problems, her future, and the relationship of the family member to the patient.

- Identify those family members willing to be supportive of the patient through their expression of feelings concerning:
    a. The patient and her future
    b. Their ability to be supportive
    c. The resources they would need to be supportive (for example, a mother with young children may be willing to assist her mother with her activities of daily living if child care is available)
- Provide a place for family members to meet and discuss the future where the patient cannot hear their discussions.
- Invite the family members who will be participating in the patient's care to care planning conferences.
- If the patient will require extensive care by family members, provide respite for care givers.
- Inform family members of changes in the patient's status.
- Crisis intervention.
- Provide orientation to resources the family can obtain for comfort in the health care facility.
- Teach family stress reduction and relaxation exercises.
- Refer to agency, community, state, and federally funded resources.

Now, identify the interventions related to the sixth goal: *The patient and/or family will understand how to implement the patient's plan of care*:

- Teach the patient/family interventions needed to
    a. Control pain, decrease anxiety, and increase relaxation
    b. Assist the patient with changes in lifestyle/activities
    c. Maintain the patient's independence and control
- Teach the patient and her family the side effects of therapy and the observations to be reported to the health team.

Lastly, identify the interventions related to the seventh goal: *The family will be assisted in modifying its lifestyle as needed*.

- Explain to the family the assistance the patient will require to be as independent as possible.
- Teach the family:
    a. The principles of problem solving to enable them to cope with a change in their lifestyle
    b. How to identify short- and long-term goals

    c. Interventions that can be implemented to meet defined goals

    d. How to identify and use resources effectively

- Explain to the family that counseling may be needed to deal with issues related to a change in the family's lifestyle. Examples include:

    a. Time required to assist the patient with plan of care

    b. Assistance with mobility

    c. Possible job modifications (transportation, special equipment)

    d. Financial needs related to the patient's therapy and future

    e. Family relationships—support and conflicts

    f. Availability of family members to be assistive

    g. Prognosis

Before proceeding to the next step, compare the interventions you have written with the goals to ensure that you have not omitted any interventions.

When you have identified all the interventions pertinent to each goal, proceed to step 5.

STEP 5
Identify the Observations Related to the Patient's Responses and the Patient's Progress

Each member of the health team needs to identify the observations that must be made to determine the patient's responses to the interventions and the patient's progress.

Every clinician should examine each goal and ask:

- What do I need to observe to identify the patient's progress toward the goals?

Each clinician should examine each intervention and ask:

- What observations must I make to monitor the patient's responses to therapy and care?

The observations related to the patient's progress toward the goals and the patient's responses to therapy and care are:

Goal 1 *The patient will be able to control her pain.*

- Observe the patient's responses to each of the interventions employed to:

    a. Reduce pain

    b. Assist the patient to decrease anxiety and increase relaxation

Note: The specific observations to be made will be determined by the interventions to be implemented. For example, for each intervention/ therapy, observe for:

    a. Side effects/effectiveness

    b. Impact of therapy on the patient's activities

    c. Patient's ability to implement interventions to control pain

- Observe the patient's ability to complete her daily schedule.

Goal 2 *The patient will be able to identify the factors, situations, or persons that increase, precipitate, or decrease her pain.*

- Observe the patient's responses to situations, factors, and persons in her environment.

- Observe the patient's responses to interventions that modify or eliminate situations, factors, and persons in the environment that increase or precipitate pain.

Goal 3 *The patient will be able to pursue or modify her prior lifestyle before the pain began to meet her present needs.*

- Observe the patient's ability to do activities related to her lifestyle prior to her pain.

- Observe the patient's interaction with members of her family, friends, co-workers, etc.

- Observe the patient's progress:

    a. Defining goals

    b. Using resources needed to implement goals

    c. Learning new methods of coping

- Observe the patient to identify the degree of independence in relation to goals.

- Observe the patient's willingness to participate in the interventions on her plan of care.

Goal 4 *The patient will not experience preventable side effects of therapy or complications.*

- Observe the patient for:

    a. Side effects/effectiveness of each intervention/therapy

    b. Complications related to:
      1. Pain
      2. Cause of pain
      3. Therapy

Goal 5 *The family will receive the assistance needed to support the patient.*

- Observe family members' interactions with each other and the patient.
- Observe each family member's participation in family planning conferences.

Goal 6 *The patient and/or family will understand how to implement the patient's plan of care on discharge.*

- Observe the patient's and each family member's responses to teaching.
- Observe the patient's and each family member's skill in implementing interventions and use of equipment.

Goal 7 *The family will be assisted in modifying its lifestyle as needed.*

- Observe the family's progress:
  a. Defining goals
  b. Using resources needed to implement goals
  c. Learning new methods of coping
- Observe each family member's willingness to participate in the interventions on the patient's plan of care.

When the health team has finished identifying all the observations, go on to step 6.

STEP 6
Specify When Each Intervention and Observation Needs to Be Done

After you have identified the essential interventions and observations, you need to specify *when* each should be done. Think about each of the interventions and answer this question:

- *How frequently* does this intervention need to be done to achieve the goals/outcome standards?

For some goals, this question is more appropriate:

- *When* does this intervention need to be done to meet the goals/outcome standards?

This question may also be useful:

- *How long* must this intervention be done to achieve the goals/outcome standards?

Ask the following questions about each observation:

- *How frequently* does each observation need to be made in order to identify:
    a. the patient's responses to each intervention?
    b. the patient's progress toward the goals/outcome standards?
- *How long* does each observation need to be done to identify:
    a. the patient's responses each intervention?
    b. the patient's progress toward the goals/outcome standards?
- *When* does each observation need to be done to identify:
    a. the patient's responses to each intervention?
    b. the patient's progress toward the goals/outcome standards?

The frequency of all the interventions and observations in the example of *Chronic Pain* is dependent on the patient's needs as well as the combination of specific interventions selected. When interventions are implemented in a close time sequence with each other, the frequency of implementing one intervention may be modified in relation to other interventions for efficiency in providing care and to ensure the patient obtains adequate rest.

Now study each goal and identify *when* the interventions and observations should be done to ensure positive outcomes for the patient:

Goal 1 *The patient will be able to control her pain.*

During assessment, identify the patient's perception of pain control.

- Explore the interventions used by the patient in the past and her evaluation of their effectiveness.*
- After the care plan has been designed, assist the patient to implement interventions that reduce pain and are congruent with the patient's cultural and religious beliefs.*

When the patient is experiencing anxiety, help the patient implement interventions that decrease anxiety and increase relaxation:

- Assist the patient with her activities *as needed.*
- Time and adjust activities to allow for optimal pain relief.*
- Schedule/modify activities to allow for adequate rest and sleep without interference with pain control schedule.*

- Observe the patient's responses to each of the interventions* used to:
  a. Reduce pain
  b. Assist the patient to decrease anxiety and increase relaxation

(The frequency of observations related to each intervention are defined when specific interventions have been identified for a patient.)

- Observe the patient's ability to complete her daily schedule.*

*Daily during patient contact, at each home visit, or during an appointment at a community agency.

Goal 2 *The patient will be able to identify the factors, situations, or persons that increase, precipitate, or decrease pain.*

- Ask the patient to identify the factors, situations, or persons in her environment that increase, precipitate, or decrease her pain (until they all have been identified).*

- Assist the patient to modify or eliminate those situations, factors, or persons that increase or precipitate her pain (after they have been identified).*

- Teach patient how to modify or eliminate those activities, factors, or persons in her environment that increase or precipitate pain (after they have been identified).*

- *When the patient is experiencing pain*, observe the patient's responses to situations, factors, or persons in her environment.

- *During and after the interventions*, observe the patient's responses to interventions that modify or eliminate situations, factors, or persons in the environment that increase or precipitate pain.

*Daily during patient contact, at each home visit, or an appointment at a community agency.

Goal 3 *The patient will be able to pursue or modify her prior lifestyle before the pain began to meet her present needs.*

- *After the pain is controlled*, interview the patient regarding her lifestyle prior to her pain.

- *After the pain is controlled*, assist the patient in comparing her lifestyle prior to her pain with her present ability to function and identify the modifications, if any, that need to be made to meet her present needs.

- Assist the patient in expressing feelings *when needed*.

- Teach problem solving in relation to modifying her lifestyle prior to pain to meet current needs *as soon as the patient can focus on non-pain topics* (when modification is needed).
- Teach the patient how to set goals that are realistic *as soon as the patient can focus on non-pain topics*.
- Assist the patient in identifying resources/supportive persons that can be assistive to her *when needed*.
- Encourage use of a support system—e.g., family, spiritual adviser, *when needed*.
- Counsel *as needed*.
- Provide positive reinforcement for achievements *at all times*.
- Identify the patient's needs for assistive devices *when needed*.
- Observe the patient's ability to do activities related to her lifestyle prior to her pain.*
- *During the interaction*, observe the patient's interaction with members of her family, friends, co-workers, etc.
- Observe the patient's progress:*
  a. Defining goals
  b. Using resources needed to implement goals
  c. Learning new methods of coping
- Observe the patient to identify the degree of independence in relation to goals.*

Observe the patient's willingness to participate in the interventions on her plan of care.*

*Daily, during patient contact, at each home visit, or during an appointment at a community agency.

Goal 4 *The patient will not experience preventable side effects of therapy or complications.*

- *During implementation of interventions and teaching sessions with the patient and/or family*, teach the patient and her family:
  a. Side effects of therapy
  b. Observations that should be reported to the health team
- *At all times*, observe the patient for:
  a. Side effects/effectiveness of each intervention/therapy

b. Complications related to:
   1. Pain
   2. Cause of pain
   3. Therapy

Goal 5 *The family will receive the assistance needed to support the patient.*

- Listen to each family member's perception of the patient's problems, her future, and the relationship of the family member to the patient.*
- Identify those family members willing to be supportive of the patient through the family members' expression of their feelings concerning:
   a. The patient and her future
   b. Their perceived ability to be supportive to the patient
   c. The resources they would need to be supportive (for example, a mother with young children might be willing to assist her mother with her Activities of Daily Living if child care is available)
- Provide a place for family members to meet and discuss the future where the patient cannot hear their discussions.*
- Invite the family members who will be participating in the patient's care to care planning conferences.*

*When the patient's plan of care is designed, the planning of family conferences/meetings with family members must be realistic in relation to when it is possible to meet with them.

- If the patient will require extensive care by family members, *the plan of care should include methods of providing respite for care givers and a time frame for the methods to be implemented.*
- Inform family members of changes in the patient's status *when changes occur.*
- Crisis intervention *when needed.*
- Provide for orientation to the resources the family can obtain for comfort in the health care facility *when the patient is admitted to the health care facility and when the family needs additional resources.*
- Teach family stress reduction and relaxation exercises *when needed.*
- Refer to agency, community, state, and federally funded resources *when needed.*
- *Observe family members' interactions with each other and the patient.*
- Observe each family member's participation *during family planning conferences.*

Goal 6 *The patient and/or family will understand how to implement the patient's plan of care on discharge.*

- Teach the patient/family interventions needed to:*
    a. Control pain, decrease anxiety, and increase relaxation
    b. Assist the patient with changes in lifestyle/activities
    c. Maintain the patient's independence and control

- Teach the patient and her family the side effects of therapy and the observations to be reported to the health team.*
- Observe the patient's and each family member's responses to teaching.*
- Observe the patient's and each family member's skill in implementing interventions and use of equipment.*

*During implementation of interventions and teaching sessions with the patient and/or family.

Note: After the content to be taught has been identified, the topics to be taught need to be sequenced. The patient/family members cannot focus on everything at once. The patient/family members will need written instructional materials to take with them at discharge.

Goal 7 *The family will be assisted in modifying its lifestyle as needed.*

- Explain to the family the assistance the patient will require to be as independent as possible as soon as the needs are identified.

- Teach the family members the principles of problem solving to enable them to cope with a change in their lifestyle.

- *During conferences and interactions with family members,*
    a. Observe the family's progress:
        1. Using resources needed to implement goals
        2. Learning new methods of coping
    b. Observe each family member's willingness to participate in the interventions on the patient's plan of care.

A teaching plan will be included in the plan of care. The patient and family will be taught after their needs have been assessed and when they are ready for teaching.

After you have specified a time for the implementation of all the interventions and observations, you have developed process standards.

STEP 7
Combine the Process Standards in a Logical Order

There are various ways to combine process standards for a unit of care. If several standards need to be implemented concurrently they can be grouped together. Listing the standards in the chronological order of their use is another technique for combining standards. Also, the standards can be combined by health discipline. After you select those standards that will be implemented for patients experiencing *Chronic Pain* at your health agency, combine the standards as your health team will use them.

Unit of Care

Health Problem: Chronic pain

Goals and Process Standards

Goal 1 *The patient will be able to control her pain.*

- *During assessment*, identify the patient's perception of pain control.
- Explore the interventions used by the patient in the past and her evaluation of their effectiveness.*
- After the care plan has been designed, assist the patient to implement interventions that reduce pain and are congruent with the patient's cultural and religious beliefs.*
- *When the patient is experiencing anxiety*, assist the patient to implement interventions that decrease anxiety and increase relaxation:
- Assist the patient with her activities *as needed*.
- Time and adjust activities to allow for optimal pain relief.*
- Schedule/modify activities to allow for adequate rest and sleep without interference with pain control schedule.*
- Observe the patient's responses to each of the interventions employed to:*
    a. Reduce pain
    b. Assist the patient in decreasing anxiety and increasing relaxation

(The frequency of observations related to each intervention are defined when specific interventions have been identified for a patient).

- Observe the patient's ability to complete her daily schedule.*

*Daily during patient contact, at each home visit, or during an appointment at a community agency.

Goal 2 *The patient will be able to identify the factors, situations, or persons that increase, precipitate, or decrease pain.*

- Ask the patient to identify the situations, factors, or persons in her environment that increase, precipitate, or decrease her pain.*
- Assist the patient to modify or eliminate those situations, factors, or persons that increase or precipitate her pain.*
- Teach patient how to modify or eliminate those activities, factors or persons in her environment that increase or precipitate pain.*
- *When the patient is experiencing pain*, observe the patient's responses to situations, factors, or persons in her environment.
- *During and after the interventions have been implemented*, observe the patient's responses to interventions that modify or eliminate situations, factors, or persons in the environment that increase or precipitate pain.

*Daily during patient contact, at each home visit, or an appointment at a community agency.

Goal 3 *The patient will be able to pursue or modify her prior lifestyle (before the pain began) to meet her present needs.*

- *After the pain is controlled*, interview the patient regarding her lifestyle prior to her pain.
- *After the pain is controlled*, assist the patient to compare her lifestyle prior to her pain with her present ability to function. Identify the modifications, if any, that need to be made to meet her present needs.
- Assist the patient to express her feelings *when needed*.
- Teach problem solving in relation to modifying her lifestyle to meet current needs *as soon as the patient can focus on non-pain topics* (when modification is needed).
- Teach the patient how to set goals that are realistic *as soon as the patient can focus on non-pain topics*.
- Assist the patient to identify resources/supportive persons that can be assistive to her *when needed*.
- Encourage use of a support system—e.g., family, spiritual adviser—*when needed*.
- Counsel *as needed*.
- Provide positive reinforcement for achievements *at all times*.

- Identify the patient's needs for assistive devices *when needed.*
- Observe the patient's ability to do activities related to her lifestyle prior to her pain.*
- Observe the patient's interaction with members of her family, friends, co-workers, etc.*
- Observe the patient's progress:*
  a. Defining goals
  b. Using resources needed to implement goals
  c. Learning new methods of coping
- Observe the patient to identify the degree of independence in relation to goals.*
- Observe the patient's willingness to participate in the interventions on her plan of care.*

*Daily during patient contact, at each home visit, or an appointment at a community agency.

Goal 4 *The patient will not experience preventable side effects of therapy or complications.*

- *During implementation of interventions and teaching sessions with the patient and/or family,* teach the patient and her family:
  a. Side effects of therapy
  b. Observations that should be reported to the health team
- *At all times,* observe the patient for:
  a. Side effects/effectiveness of each intervention/therapy
  b. Complications related to:
    1. Pain
    2. Cause of pain
    3. Therapy

Goal 5 *The family will receive the assistance needed to support the patient.*

- Listen to each family member's perception of the patient's problems, her future, and the relationship of the family member to the patient.*
- Identify those family members willing to be supportive of the patient through the family members' expression of their feelings concerning:*
  a. The patient and her future
  b. Their perceived ability to be supportive to the patient

    c. The resources they would need to be supportive (for example, a mother with young children might be willing to assist her mother with her Activities of Daily Living if child care is available)

- Provide a place for family members to meet and discuss the future where the patient cannot hear their discussions.*
- Invite the family members who will be participating in the patient's care to care planning conferences.*
- If the patient will require extensive care by family members, provide respite for care givers and a time frame for the methods to be implemented.
- Inform family members of changes in the patient's status *when changes occur.*
- Crisis intervention *when needed.*
- Provide for orientation to resources available to the family in the health care facility *when the patient is admitted to the health care facility* and *when the family needs additional resources.*
- Teach family stress reduction and relaxation exercises *when needed.*
- Refer to agency, community, state, and federally funded resources *when needed.*
- Observe family members' interactions with each other and the patient.
- Observe each family member's participation during family planning conferences.

*When the interventions are implemented as defined in each patient's plan of care. Planning must be realistic in relation to meeting with family members.

Goal 6 *The patient and/or family will understand how to implement the patient's plan of care.*

- Teach the patient/family interventions needed to:*
  - a. Control pain, decrease anxiety, and increase relaxation
  - b. Assist the patient with changes in lifestyle/activities
  - c. Maintain the patient's independence and control
- Teach the patient and her family the side effects of therapy and the observations to be reported to the health team.*
- Observe the patient's and each family member's responses to teaching.*
- Observe the patient's and each family member's skill in implementing interventions and use of equipment.*

*During implementation of the interventions and teaching sessions with the patient and/or family.

Goal 7 *The family will be assisted in modifying its lifestyle as needed.*

- Explain to the family the assistance the patient will require to be as independent as possible.*
- Teach the family:*
    a. The principles of problem solving to enable them to cope with a change in their lifestyle
    b. How to identify short- and long-term goals
    c. Interventions that can be implemented to meet defined goals
- Observe the family's progress:*
    a. Defining goals
    b. Using resources needed to implement goals
    c. Learning new methods of coping
- Observe each family member's willingness to participate in the interventions on the patient's plan of care.*

*During contact with the family in an inpatient setting, home visit, or planned visits to the community health agency.[1][2][3]

STEP 8
Eliminate Suggestions and Rationale from the Process Standards You Have Written

Suggestions and rationale are sometimes mistakenly identified as process standards. Read section 5 of chapter 2 to determine whether any of the process standards you have written are really suggestions or rationales. Eliminate any suggestions and statements of rationale from your list of process standards. Then go on to step 9.

STEP 9
Identify Which Health Discipline Will Be Responsible for Implementing Each Intervention and Observation

After the process standards have been identified for a health problem/patient care need, the health team should decide which member should implement each of the interventions and observations. The clinician who should collect the data can be identified based on the following criteria:

1. The clinician who has the skills to implement interventions and/or make observations
2. The clinician(s) who will be in the health agency when interventions should be implemented/observations need to be made
3. The staffing of the clinicians in a specific health discipline is ample enough to do the work

After each process standard specify the name of the health team member who will assume responsibility for obtaining data on that outcome; then proceed to the next step.

STEP 10
Establish the Validity of the Process Standards

Although you have developed process standards, they are not ready for implementation. Refer to chapter 5 to establish the validity of the process standards you have written.

You have completed the section on how to write process standards for an interdisciplinary unit of care. Now you may proceed to the next section, "Writing Outcome Standards for an Interdisciplinary Unit of Care," or you may want to begin reading chapter 5, "Writing Content Standards."

SECTION 4
Writing Outcome Standards for Interdisciplinary Units of Care

The evaluation of the patient's progress toward the goals of her plan of care using patient outcomes is vital to ensure that the interventions/observations being implemented by clinicians from multiple health disciplines are producing positive outcomes for patients. The outcomes need to be written so that:

1. Those evaluating the patient's status understand what observations to make
2. The patient's status is evaluated at a point in time that will provide the clinicians with information to identify the patient's progress, prevent complications, and provide the information needed to keep the patient's plan of care current

Before writing the outcomes for interdisciplinary units of care, the clinicians of each health discipline should identify the patient outcomes related to the interventions implemented by their discipline. Then, when the health team meets to develop interdisciplinary units of care, the outcomes from all disciplines can be integrated into the unit of care and the responsibility for evaluating the outcomes can be assigned. This assignment of responsibility for data collection is important to prevent unnecessary duplication in data collection.

Before members of the health team begin writing outcome standards, the group must agree on the approach to assigning titles of the units of care. This is important because the title provides a mental picture of one or more health dimensions of the patient and leads the health professional to identify the goals and then the outcome standards. The most common approach used for identifying titles for units of care is either as a health problem or patient care need. A **health problem/patient care need** can be defined as a collection of signs and symptoms that, taken together, constitute a picture of ill health or health care required by the patient. The health problem/patient care need is expressed in a word or phrase that triggers in the mind of the clinician a picture of the health problem/patient care need and the interventions pertinent to its resolution.

METHOD

The ten steps in writing process standards for an interdisciplinary unit of care are:

1. Define the unit of care.
2. Specify the time frame.
3. Identify the goals of care.
4. Identify the positive outcomes that are expected to occur.
5. Identify the negative outcomes that can be avoided.
6. Specify when you expect each outcome to occur.
7. Clarify the description of the expected outcomes.
8. Combine the outcome standards in a logical order.
9. Identify which health discipline will be responsible for collecting data on each outcome.
10. Establish the validity of the outcome standards.

STEP 1
Define the Unit of Care

The first step in writing outcome standards is to create a name or title for the unit of care. This title must be understood by *every* member of the health team. As the team discusses the name, each member should decide whether the unit of care can be broken into smaller health problems/patient care needs. (You may want to review the example related to assigning titles to units of care in section 1 of this chapter.)

To assist in identifying units of care, review the plans of care developed for patients in past planning meetings. Or, obtain a list of the problems/needs usually presented by patients admitted to your agency. It is recommended that you begin with problems/needs of patients most frequently seen or the problems/needs where interdisciplinary cooperation is vital to achieve positive outcomes for patients. Also, review the requirements from accrediting or reimbursing agencies to ensure that you have written standards for those health problems/needs that are expected by these agencies.

The unit of care that will be used as the example for writing interdisciplinary outcome standards is the *Patient in Chronic Pain*. Chronic pain can be defined as the discomfort experienced by a person over a period of time such that the end to the pain cannot be identified. Chronic pain is further defined by the patient's health status identified during the initial assessment. The pain is severe enough that it affects the patient's health status in bodily areas not affected by the pain and affects the patient's lifestyle and relationships with other people.

After you have selected a title for the unit of care, go on to step 2.

STEP 2
Specify the Time Frame

Some units of care require a time frame because the goals and interventions as well as the outcomes change as the patient progresses through phases of illness and treatment. For example, some of the goals and interventions are the same for patients experiencing *Potential for Thrombophlebitis, Acute Thrombophlebitis* while the patient is on bedrest and her leg is immobilized and *Thrombophlebitis* during the *Ambulatory* and *Health Teaching* phases of this health problem.

To identify whether a time frame is needed for this unit of care, ask yourself:

- At what identifiable time periods will the patient require a different unit of care?
- When must I change the care as the patient's health status changes?

In our example, the time frame for the unit of care *Chronic Pain* is defined in the title. The time frame is when the patient is experiencing pain over an extended time period. The pain is not being controlled by the patient and is impairing the quality of her lifestyle and her ability to function. The patient's responses to the chronic pain may also be affecting her family's lifestyle. Further specification of a time frame for this unit of care could be:

    a. Post-injury, when the patient is receiving therapy on an outpatient basis to rebuild muscle strength

    b. During rehabilitation, after a spinal cord injury when the patient has spastic paralysis

After you have thought about whether a time frame is needed for this unit of care, proceed to the next step.

STEP 3
Identify the Goals of Care

The goals provide the framework for writing the outcomes of care. A **goal** is an explicit statement describing exactly what you plan to accomplish with the care. As you think about a health problem/patient care need and its time frame, ask yourself:

- What can be done to help a patient having this health problem/need?
- What interventions implemented by members of the health team can eliminate or reduce the impact of this health problem/patient care need?

The goals for the *Patient in Chronic Pain* are:

- The patient will be able to control her pain.
- The patient will be able to identify the factors, situations, or persons that increase, precipitate, or decrease her pain.
- The patient will be able to pursue or modify her lifestyle before the pain began to meet her present needs.
- The patient will not experience preventable side effects of therapy or complications.
- The family will receive assistance to support the patient.

- The patient and/or family will understand how to implement the patient's plan of care.
- The family will be assisted in modifying its lifestyle as needed.

Note: When the goals are individualized for a specific patient, the exact date for the achievement of the goal must be specified.

After you have identified the goals, proceed to step 4.

STEP 4
Identify the Positive Outcomes That Are Expected to Occur

You may wish to reread "Types of Positive Outcomes" and "The Expected Outcome" in section 1, chapter 3 before proceeding with this step. To identify the positive outcomes of the care for this patient, ask yourself:

- What positive outcomes can I expect if the interventions related to this goal are implemented as planned?

Positive outcomes are easily identified if the goals of the unit of care are well-defined. Thus, if you have difficulty answering this question, review the goals you have written and revise them as needed. Now identify the outcomes related to each goal.

Consider the first goal: *The patient will be able to control her pain.* Ask yourself:

- What positive outcomes can I expect if the interventions related to this goal are implemented as planned?

The positive outcomes related to this goal are:

- The patient is pain free, or
- The patient expresses that she can control her pain.
- The patient is able to do her daily activities without pain (with assistance as needed).
- The patient is not experiencing increased anxiety.

The second goal, *the patient will be able to identify the factors, situations, or persons that decrease pain*, will result in the following positive outcomes:

- The patient can identify factors, situations, or persons that assist in *decreasing* her pain.

The third goal, *the patient will be able to pursue or modify her lifestyle before the pain began to meet her present needs*, if met, will result in these outcomes:

- The patient can describe/explain the differences in her ability to function prior to the pain as compared to the present.
- The patient's physiologic status has returned to pre-pain levels and/or the patient expresses satisfaction with her health status.
- The patient can focus on non-pain topics.
- The patient can identify resources/supportive persons that are helpful to her.
- The patient is using resources and/or consultations, when appropriate, to meet her needs.
- When the patient has had to modify her lifestyle, she expresses that she received the assistance, support, or teaching needed to create the changes in her lifestyle.
- The patient can explain the principles of problem solving in relation to modifying her lifestyle.
- The patient can formulate realistic short-term and long-term goals related to modifying her lifestyle.
- The patient can explain interventions to be implemented to meet defined goals.
- The patient has received the assistive devices she needs to maintain her independence.
- The patient expresses satisfaction with her orientation to the resources she has needed in the health care agency. If not, additional orientation is being implemented for her.
- The patient expresses satisfaction with the clinicians' willingness to listen to her perceptions and contributions to her plan of care.
- The patient expresses satisfaction with the assistance she has received or is receiving. If not, a health team member is intervening into the cause of the dissatisfaction.

The outcomes for the fourth goal are found in the next step. Identify the negative outcomes that can be avoided.

The outcomes for the fifth goal, *the family will receive assistance to support the patient*, are:

- The family expresses satisfaction with its orientation to the resources it has needed in the health care agency.
- The family expresses satisfaction with the clinicians' willingness to listen to its perceptions and contributions to the patient's plan of care.

- The family members who are willing to support the patient express satisfaction with the assistance they have received or are receiving.

The sixth goal, *the patient and/or family will understand how to implement the patient's plan of care*, will result in the following outcomes:

- The patient and family can explain/demonstrate how to implement each intervention/therapy to:
  a. Control pain
  b. Decrease anxiety
  c. Increase relaxation
  d. Make changes in the patient's lifestyle/activities
  e. Maintain the patient's independence and control

For example, the patient and her family need to:
  a. Know how the patient should take her medications
  b. Know activities the patient can do without increasing pain
  c. Have assistance from others needed by the patient

- If she is not correctly implementing one or more interventions, the patient and/or family member is working with (insert name of health professional or agency where the patient has been referred) to improve the technique.

The seventh goal, *the family will be assisted in modifying its lifestyle as needed*, if met, will result in these outcomes:

- The family members express that they have received or are receiving assistance in modifying their lifestyle when needed.
- The family members can identify resources/supportive persons that are helpful to them.
- The family members are using resources and/or consultations, when appropriate, to meet their needs.
- The family members can explain the principles of problem solving in relation to modifying their lifestyle.
- The family members can formulate short-term and long-term goals related to modifying their lifestyle.
- The family members can explain interventions to be implemented to meet defined goals.

After you have identified all the positive outcomes for every goal, review all the goals and outcomes together to ascertain whether you have identified all the positive outcomes. Then proceed to the next step.

STEP 5
Identify the Negative Outcomes That Can Be Avoided

Before proceeding, you may wish to review "Types of Negative Outcomes" in section 1, chapter 3. To identify the negative outcomes preventable with excellent care, ask yourself:

- What negative outcomes can be avoided if the care related to this goal is implemented as planned?

There are two goals that relate to negative outcomes:

1. The outcomes for the fourth goal, *the patient will not experience preventable side effects of therapy or complications,* are:
   - The patient is not experiencing undetected signs and symptoms of the side effects of therapy or complications. If any signs and symptoms are present, they have been reported to _____ (the health professional that can treat the complication).
   - If any signs and symptoms are present, interventions have been initiated to treat the side effect/complication. (The specific outcomes for this goal cannot be defined until the interventions/therapy have been identified.)
2. The second goal, *the patient will be able to identify the factors, situations, or persons that increase or precipitate pain,* will result in the following positive outcomes:
   - The patient can identify factors, situations, or persons that assist in *increasing* or *precipitating* her pain.
   - The patient can demonstrate/explain how to modify or eliminate those factors/situations/persons that assist in *increasing* or *precipitating* her pain.

All negative outcomes are written so that a "yes" response to the standard means the patient experienced a positive outcome. This is done to ensure clarity during the evaluation of the care related to the outcome.

After you have written all the negative outcomes as outcome statements, go on to step 6.

STEP 6
Specify When You Expect Each Outcome to Occur

Before proceeding with this step, you may wish to review "When the Outcome Will Occur" in section 1 of chapter 3. Now review each of the following outcomes and ask yourself:

- When can I expect this outcome to occur?

Each goal is listed with its outcomes. "When the outcome will occur" is in italics.

Goal 1 *The patient will be able to control her pain.*

- The patient is pain free,* or
- The patient expresses that she can control her pain.*
- After the patient's pain has been controlled, the patient is able to do her daily activities without pain (with assistance as needed).*

Within _____ hours/days or _____ home visits or _____ appointments at a community agency.

- At all times the patient is not experiencing increased anxiety.

Goal 2 *The patient will be able to identify the factors/situations that decrease pain.*

- The patient can identify factors, situations, or persons that assist in *decreasing* her pain.*
- The patient can identify factors, situations, or persons that assist in *increasing* or *precipitating* her pain.*

Within _____ hours/days or _____ home visits or _____ appointments at a community agency.

After the factors, situations, or persons have been identified, the patient can demonstrate/explain how to modify or eliminate those factors, situations, or persons that assist in *increasing* or *precipitating* her pain *within days or _____ home visits or _____ appointments at a community agency.*

Goal 3 *The patient will be able to pursue or modify her lifestyle before the pain began to meet her present needs.*

- The patient can describe/explain the differences in her ability to function prior to the pain as compared to the present.*

- The patient's physiologic status has returned to pre-pain levels and/or the patient expresses satisfaction with her health status.*
- The patient can focus on non-pain topics.*

Within _____ hours/days or _____ home visits or _____ appointments at a community agency.

After the patient is able to control her pain:

- The patient can identify resources/supportive persons that are helpful to her.*
- The patient is using resources and/or consultations, when appropriate to meet her needs.*
- When the patient has had to modify her lifestyle, she expresses she received the assistance/support/teaching needed to create the changes in her lifestyle.*
- The patient can explain the principles of problem solving in relation to modifying her lifestyle.*
- The patient can formulate realistic short-term and long-term goals related to modifying her lifestyle.*
- The patient can explain interventions to be implemented to meet defined goals.*
- *Within 24 hours after the need for a device has been identified*, the patient has received the assistive devices she needs to maintain her independence.
- *During and after the orientation* the patient expresses satisfaction with her orientation to the resources she has needed in the health care agency. If not, additional orientation is being implemented for her.[+]
- *At all times* the patient expresses satisfaction with the clinicians' willingness to listen to her perceptions and contributions to her plan of care.[+]
- *At all times* the patient expresses satisfaction with the assistance she has received or is receiving. If not, a health team member is intervening into the cause of the dissatisfaction.[+]

Within _____ hours/days or _____ home visits or _____ appointments at a community agency.

[+]Patient satisfaction outcomes.

Goal 4 *The patient will not experience preventable side effects of therapy or complications.*

- *At all times* the patient is not experiencing undetected signs and symptoms of complications. If any signs and symptoms are present, they have been reported to _____ (the health professional that can treat the side effect/complication).
- *At all times*, if any signs and symptoms are present, interventions have been initiated to treat the side effect/complication.

Goal 5 *The family will receive assistance to support the patient.*

- *During and after the orientation* family members express satisfaction with their orientation to the resources they have needed in the health care agency. If not, additional orientation is being implemented for family members. +
- *At all times* family members express satisfaction with the clinicians' willingness to listen to their perceptions and contributions to the patient's plan of care. +
- *At all times* the family members who are willing to support the patient express satisfaction with the assistance they have received or are receiving. If not, a health team member is intervening into the cause of the dissatisfaction. +

+Family satisfaction outcomes.

Goal 6 *The patient and/or family will understand how to implement the patient's plan of care.*

- The patient and family can explain/demonstrate how to implement each intervention/therapy to:*
  - a. Control pain
  - b. Decrease anxiety
  - c. Increase relaxation
  - d. Make changes in the patient's lifestyle/activities
  - e. Maintain the patient's independence and control
- If the patient or family member is not correctly implementing one or more interventions, they are working with _____ (insert name of health professional or agency where the patient has been referred) to improve the technique.*

*Patient/family members are interviewed during several days or several appointments at the community agency or during several home visits before the patient is discharged from the agency. This interview is conducted to identify the level of knowledge/skill of those being taught the interventions that must be continued after discharge. If, at the time of evaluation, the patient/family member can not demonstrate or explain what they need to do after discharge, the patient's discharge plan must contain resources that will continue the teaching post discharge. Also, the patient/family members should receive information that they can refer to after discharge related to interventions and therapy they must continue.

Goal 7 *The family will be assisted in modifying its lifestyle as needed.*

- The family members express that they have received or are receiving assistance in modifying their lifestyle when needed.*
- The family members can identify resources/supportive persons that are helpful to them.*
- The family members are using resources and/or consultations, when appropriate, to meet their needs.*
- The family members can explain the principles of problem solving in relation to modifying their lifestyle.*
- The family members can formulate short-term and long-term goals related to modifying their lifestyle.*
- The family members can explain interventions to be implemented to meet defined goals.*

Within _____ hours/days or _____ home visits or _____ appointments at a community agency.

In many of the outcomes in this example you have seen the phrase "Within _____ hours/days or _____ home visits or _____ appointments at a community agency." If the patient is in an inpatient setting, the phrase "within hour/days" is appropriate. When the patient is receiving therapy from a community agency, the outcomes would be evaluated during an appointment to a community agency or during a home visit.

When outcomes relate to provision of comfort for the patient/family, patient/family satisfaction, and prevention of complications, the "when" is *at all times.* When the phrase *at all times* is attached to an outcome, the positive outcome should be present at any time you are with the patient.

Note: When the outcomes are individualized for a specific patient, the exact date for the achievement of the outcomes must be defined.

When you have completed this step, proceed to step 7.

STEP 7
Clarify the Description of the Expected Outcomes

As you may remember, each outcome statement should be written as specifically as is needed by every staff member implementing the care. The following outcomes contain the necessary specification that might need to be included for staff to evaluate the care given using these outcomes:

- *Before discharge*, the patient's physiologic status has returned to pre-pain levels and/or the patient expresses satisfaction with health status.

Some examples of patient's functions that can be affected by chronic pain and/or the therapy/interventions to control pain are:

a. Fatigue
b. Sleep pattern
c. Nutritional status
d. Weight
e. Energy level
f. Activity level
g. Bowel pattern
h. Level of decision making
i. Activities of Daily Living
j. Menstrual cycle
k. Libido
l. Anxiety
m. Memory
n. Level of alertness

This list is an example of patient functions that can be affected by chronic pain and/or the treatment of it. These items remind each health professional to obtain a total evaluation of the impact of the chronic pain and the treatment of it when they are evaluating the patient's progress.

- *Before discharge*, the patient and family can explain/demonstrate how to implement each intervention/therapy to:
  a. Control pain
  b. Decrease anxiety
  c. Increase relaxation
  d. Make changes in lifestyle/activities
  e. Maintain the patient's independence and control

The interventions to be taught to the patient will be defined as the interventions for a specific patient are defined. But, for example, the patient will need to know:

a. How to take each medication: when to take them, what symptoms to report to the health team, and any special drug/food interactions to avoid

b. Pattern of rest and activity: when to take rest periods and the length of rest periods

c. Activities she can do without increasing pain and activities to avoid in her schedule

d. Assistance required of family: if the patient can no longer do the functions/chores that are meaningful for family members, who will do them

In the following outcome, it is essential that every member of the staff providing care to this patient know what signs and symptoms indicate a complication or an untoward effect of the therapy or intervention. Thus you may want to identify specific observations to be made for these signs/symptoms when the patient's plan of care is designed. It is also important to identify which member of the health team will be responsible for intervening so that time is not lost intervening in a possible or actual complication.

• The patient is not experiencing undetected signs and symptoms of complications. If any signs and symptoms are present, it has been reported to _____ (the health professional that can treat the complication).

• If any signs and symptoms are present, interventions have been initiated to treat the side effect/complication.

You will note that some of these outcomes contain the phrase "it has been reported to the health professional who can intervene in the situation." This phrase is a qualifying statement that defines the responsibility of the health professional who can intervene if the outcome is becoming negative. It is important to identify what health discipline should intervene if outcomes are becoming negative so there is no time lost in intervention. For more information on qualifying statements, read chapter 6, section 1.

STEP 8
Combine the Outcome Standards in a Logical Order

The finished unit of care contains a title for the unit of care, lists its goals, and combines the outcome standards in a way health professionals will implement them. There are various ways to combine standards for a unit of care. If several standards need to be implemented concurrently, they can be grouped together. Listing the standards in the chronological order of their use is another technique for combining standards. Also, the standards can be combined by health discipline. After you select those standards that will be implemented for patients at your health agency, combine the standards as your health team will use them.

Before beginning this step, think about how the standards you have written will be implemented. A suggested way to combine the standards for this unit of care is presented below.

Unit of Care

Health Problem: Chronic Pain

Goals and Outcome Standards

Goal 1 *The patient will be able to control her pain.*

1. The patient is pain free,* or
2. The patient expresses that she can control her pain.*
3. After the patient's pain has been controlled, the patient is able to do her daily activities without pain (with assistance as needed).*
4. At all times the patient is not experiencing increased anxiety.

*Within _____ hours/days or _____ home visits or _____ appointments at a community agency.

Goal 2 *The patient will be able to identify the factors, situations, or persons that increase, precipitate or decrease pain.*

1. The patient can identify factors, situations, or persons that assist in *decreasing* her pain.*
2. The patient can identify factors, situations, or persons that assist in *increasing* or *precipitating* her pain.*

3. After the factors, situations, or persons have been identified, the patient can demonstrate/explain how to modify or eliminate those that assist in increasing or precipitating her pain.*

Within _____ hours/days or _____ home visits or _____ appointments at a community agency.

Goal 3 *The patient will be able to pursue or modify her prior lifestyle before the pain began to meet her present needs.*

1. The patient can describe/explain the differences in her ability to function prior to the pain as compared to the present.*
2. The patient's physiological status has returned to pre-pain levels and/or the patient expresses satisfaction with her health status.*
3. The patient can focus on non-pain topics.*

After the patient is able to control her pain:

4. The patient can identify resources/supportive persons that are helpful to her.*
5. The patient is using resources and/or consultations, when appropriate to meet her needs.*
6. When the patient has had to modify her lifestyle, she expresses that she received the assistance, support, and teaching needed to create the changes in her lifestyle.*
7. The patient can explain the principles of problem solving in relation to modifying her lifestyle.*
8. The patient can formulate realistic short-term and long-term goals related to modifying her lifestyle.*
9. The patient can explain interventions to be implemented to meet defined goals.*
10. *Within 24 hours after the need for a device has been identified,* the patient has received the assistive devices she needs to maintain her independence.
11. *During and after the orientation* the patient expresses satisfaction with her orientation to the resources she has needed in the health care agency. If not, additional orientation is being implemented for her.
12. *At all times* the patient expresses satisfaction with the clinicians' willingness to listen to her perceptions and contributions to her plan of care.

13. *At all times* the patient expresses satisfaction with the assistance she has received or is receiving. If not, a health team member is intervening into the cause of the dissatisfaction.

*Within _____ hours/days or _____ home visits or _____ appointments at a community agency.

Goal 4 *The patient will not experience preventable side effects of therapy or complications.*

1. *At all times* the patient is not experiencing undetected signs and symptoms of complications. If any signs and symptoms are present, they have been reported to _____ (the health professional that can treat the side effect/complication).

2. *At all times*, if any signs and symptoms are present, interventions have been initiated to treat the side effect/complication.

Goal 5 *The family will receive assistance to support the patient.*

1. *During and after the orientation* family members express satisfaction with their orientation to the resources they have needed in the health care agency. If not, additional orientation is being implemented for family members.

2. *At all times* family members express satisfaction with the clinicians' willingness to listen to their perceptions and contributions to the patient's plan of care.

3. *At all times* the family members who are willing to support the patient express satisfaction with the assistance they have received or are receiving. If not, a health team member is intervening into the cause of the dissatisfaction.

Goal 6 *The patient and/or family will understand how to implement the patient's plan of care.*

1. The patient and family can explain/demonstrate how to implement each intervention/therapy to:*
   a. Control pain
   b. Decrease anxiety
   c. Increase relaxation
   d. Make changes in the patient's lifestyle/activities
   e. Maintain the patient's independence and control

2. If the patient or family member is not correctly implementing one or more interventions, they are working with _____

(insert name of health professional or agency where the patient has been referred) to improve the technique.*

*Patient/family members are interviewed during several days or during several appointments at the community agency or during several home visits before the patient is discharged from the agency to identify the level of knowledge/skill of those being taught the interventions that must be continued after discharge.

Goal 7 *The family will be assisted in modifying its lifestyle as needed.*

1. The family members express that they have received or are receiving assistance in modifying their lifestyle when needed.*
2. The family members can identify resources/supportive persons that are helpful to them.*
3. The family members are using resources and/or consultations, when appropriate, to meet their needs.*
4. The family members can explain the principles of problem solving in relation to modifying their lifestyle.*
5. The family members can formulate short-term and long-term goals related to modifying their lifestyle.*
6. The family members can explain interventions to be implemented to meet defined goals.*

Within _____ hours/days or _____ home visits or _____ appointments at a community agency.

Note: When the goals are individualized for a specific patient, the exact date for the achievement of the goal must be specified.

STEP 9
Identify Which Health Discipline Will Be Responsible for Collecting Data on Each Outcome

After the outcomes have been identified for a health problem/patient care need, the health team should decide which member of the team should collect the data related to each of the outcomes. The clinician who should collect the data can be identified based on the following criteria:

a. Implements the interventions related to the outcome
b. Is the clinician who collected similar data on the initial assessment of the patient (This is important to identify the changes in the patient from initial asssessment to the present.)

c. Has the assessment skills required to make the evaluation of the patient's status

All clinicians on the health team need to participate in the evaluation to obtain a "photograph" of the patient's need/health problems at the present time.

After each of the outcomes contains the name of the health team member who will assume responsibility for obtaining data on that outcome, proceed to the next step.

STEP 10
Establish the Validity of the Outcome Standards

Although you have developed outcome standards, they are not ready for implementation. Refer to chapter 5 to establish the validity of the outcome standards you have written.

You have completed the section on how to write outcome standards for an interdisciplinary unit of care. You may want to go back to the previous section, "Writing Process Standards for Interdisciplinary Units of Care," or, you may want to begin reading chapter 5, "Writing Content Standards."

NOTES

1. Carpenito, Lynda Juall. *Nursing diagnosis: Application to clinical practice* (4th ed.), pp. 237–245. New York: J.B. Lipincott and Co., 1992.

2. Wesorick, Bonnie. *Standards of nursing care: A model for clinical practice,* p. 215. New York: J.B. Lippincott and Co., 1990.

3. Thompson, June M., McFarland, Gertrude K., Hirsch, Jane E., Tucker, Susan M., and Bowers, Arden C. *Clinical nursing* (4th ed.), pp. 1538–1544. St. Louis: C.V. Mosby Co., 1993.

5

Writing Content Standards

Content standards contribute to positive outcomes of nursing care by defining the content of assessment. Content standards enable the nurse to provide the patient and his family with the type of information they need to prevent or cope with a health problem. Communication with patients can contain interventions for psychological and sociological patient care needs or health problems.

Content standards also must be written concerning the decisions nurses make in emergency situations. Nurses must intervene rapidly in emergency situations; thus, they must be able to evaluate the patient's situation and intevene rapidly to prevent negative outcomes for patients.

The quality of the communications between nurses and patients or other health professionals is an essential component of nursing care. Therefore, content standards need to be developed for communications nurses have with others for the benefit of the patient.

This chapter has six sections. The first three sections describe how to write standards concerning the communications with patients and their families. Writing content standards for assessment is in section 1. Writing content standards for teaching is presented in section 2. Writing content standards for therapeutic communication is the subject of section 3. Developing content standards for decision making in emergency situations is the focus of section 4. The last two sections cover the types of communication nurses have with other health professionals.

Section 5 describes how to write content standards for documentation. The method of writing content standards for reporting is explained in section 6.

The format of this chapter is similar to that of chapters 2 and 3. You can study each section independently of the others. The overall method is described, followed by a specific discussion and an example to illustrate each step. You are also provided with questions to guide you in writing the standards. Now, proceed to the section in the chapter that you want to study to learn to write content standards.

SECTION 1
Writing Content Standards for Assessment

Nurses use therapeutic communication with patients and family for the purpose of obtaining data for planning care and establishing a baseline for data collection in the future. Content standards need to be developed for all data collection tools to provide consistency from nurse to nurse in data collection. The content standards define the categories of data essential to the provision of care.

Assessments can be included with interventions and observations in units of care or a total assessment may be an entire unit of care. Thus, after you have completed the writing of all of your units of care, review the assessments you have developed in relation to:

a. The selection of units of care during care planning
b. The patient outcomes of all the units of care for reassessment and evaluation after the patient has received nursing care

There are two major types of data collection: total assessment and focused assessment. **Total assessment** can be defined as data collection concerning all characteristics of the patient and factors external to the patient that should be considered when planning and implementing nursing care.

Examples of total assessment, in addition to the admission, are the assessments that need to be made before special therapies are begun, e.g., outpatient clinic, hospice. These assessments are done to establish a baseline before the therapy and care begin and at periodic intervals during the health care. Because assessment data are a baseline for the next assessment and will be used to identify the patient's response to therapy and the patient's progress toward the patient outcomes, the categories of data in the assessment should include all the outcomes listed in the outcome standards. For example, if the quality of the breath sounds is one of the outcome standards, the patient's breath sounds should be auscultated on admission to establish a baseline and be included on every assessment that is done to identify the progress of the patient and the patient's response to therapy and care. At periodic intervals the nurse can look back at the baseline to identify whether the patient has experienced improvement in one or more dimensions of his health status. At these periodic assessments the nurse should decide if the patient's plan of care is meeting the needs of the patient or should be modified if the patient is not making satisfactory progress. There are certain common categories of data that are usually included in total assessments. These are:

- Biophysical status
- Psychosocial status
- Self-care status
- Family roles and responsibilities
- Factors affecting discharge planning
- Environmental factors
- Available resources
- Needs for education and factors affecting learning

Focused assessment is data collection related to a potential or actual patient care need or health problem. A focused assessment is needed to identify the history and characteristics of patients, as well as external factors that will provide specific data needed by the nurse for planning and evaluating interventions in a unit of care.

For example, the "Potential for Falls Assessment" is done to identify patients with those characteristics that might predispose patients to fall, while a "Skin Assessment" is done to identify the factors that might predispose the patient to skin breakdown. After assessment, the nurse can identify interventions to prevent these potential health problems from occurring. On the other hand, a "Pain Assessment" is done to identify the effectiveness of the pain interventions that are being implemented.

Focused assessments are also done before certain therapies to identify those categories of data likely to change as a result of the therapy. Examples are: chemotherapy, physical therapy, or medical procedures such as liver biopsy and thoracentesis.

METHOD

The method of writing content standards related to obtaining data from patients consists of five steps:

1. Define the patient's health situation.
2. Identify the goals of data collection.
3. Identify the items of data collection.
4. Combine the content standards in a logical order.
5. Establish the validity of the standards.

After you have completed step 5, the standards you have written will be ready for implementation. Now begin with step 1.

STEP 1
Define the Patient's Health Situation

An accurate description of the patient's health situation can help you to identify the goals of data collection. This description should be brief but must contain the detail necessary to provide a picture of a patient requiring health care. Examples of when to assess patients' health situations are:

- On admission to a health facility
- A first visit to an outpatient clinic
- A first home visit
- Teaching related to a health problem
- Before discharge planning is begun
- Updating a plan of care
- Identification of the need to prevent falls or skin breakdown

An example of a patient's health situation requiring assessment is the *Potential for Falls.*

After you have specified the patient's health situation, go on to step 2.

STEP 2
Identify the Goals of Data Collection

A major consideration in relation to the goals of data collection are the types of health services that can be provided for patients by this agency. The goals of the services may be maintenance of the patient's health or the treatment of acutely and chronically ill. Because the therapy for maintaining health is different from that for the acutely ill patient, the data that need to be collected from patients may be different. It is important that patients are not asked for information that is nonessential for the provision of services. Obtaining unnecessary information is bothersome to the patient.

You also need to determine whether the patients you are assessing require a focused or total assessment. A *total assessment* comprises *all* characteristics of the patient, while only selected categories of data are included in a *focused assessment*.

You also may want to review the definition of a goal. A **goal** is an explicit statement describing what data you want to obtain from the patient. Thus, the type of data you collect from a patient will include the nature of the patient's health situation, whether you need a focused or total assessment, and the goals for data collection.

To identify the goals, you need to answer these questions:

- What do I need to know about this patient:
- To develop his plan of care?
- To teach him what he needs to know?
- To identify a significant change in his condition?
- To prepare him for discharge?
- To identify if he needs a preventive program?

The goals for the example *Potential for Falls* are:

- To identify which patients have the potential for falling
- To identify what interventions might need to be on the patient's plan of care to prevent falling

Note: When the goals are individualized for a specific patient, the exact date for the achievement of the goals must be defined.

Now proceed to step 3.

STEP 3
Identify the Items of Data Collection

The next task is to identify the items of data to be collected. As you examine each goal, ask yourself:

- What data must I collect to design this patient's plan of care?
- What data are essential to obtain from the patient and the patient's family ?

When you have obtained answers to these questions, you will have identified the content standards for this data collection tool.

The following items should be included in a focused assessment for *Potential for Falls*.

- History of falling
- History of or current alcohol and/or drug abuse
- Poor eyesight with or without glasses
- Vertigo
- History of seizures
- Decreased level of consciousness
- Hallucinations
- Delusions
- Neurological disorders affecting coordination
- The effects of a sedative or anesthesia
- Postural hypotension
- Medication that might cause dizziness, uncoordination, confusion, delerium, postural hypotension
- Unsafe shoes/slippers
- Frequent need to urinate or defecate

All the assessment items can assist you in designing a care plan that will include interventions to prevent the patient from falling.

STEP 4
Combine the Content Standards in a Logical Order

The completed unit of care identifies the patient's health situation, lists the goals of the communication, and combines the content standards in a logical order. Review all the items of data collection for completeness and then list them in an order that is most useful to the nurses who will be implementing them. The following order is just one way the standards can be listed:

Unit of Care

Health Problem: Potential for Falls

Goals

1. To identify which patients have the potential for falling
2. To identify what interventions might need to be on the patient's plan of care to prevent falling

Note: When the goals are individualized for a specific patient, the exact date for the achievement of the goals must be defined.

Content Standards

- History of falling
- History of or current alcohol and/or drug abuse
- Poor eyesight with or without glasses
- Vertigo
- Seizures
- Agitation
- Confusion
- Decreased level of consciousness
- Hallucinations
- Delusions
- Neurological disorder affecting coordination
- The effects of a sedative or anesthesia
- Postural hypotension
- Medication that might cause dizziness, uncoordination, confusion, delirium, postural hypotension
- Unsafe shoes/slippers
- Frequent need to urinate or defecate[2]

STEP 5
Establish the Validity of the Standards

Although you have developed content standards, these standards are not necessarily valid. The standards need to be reviewed by three people knowledgeable about the data that must be collected. This step is done to ensure the content validity of the standards. After there is agreement among the experts that these are the content standards, the standards are ready for implementation. You have completed this section.

SECTION 2
Writing Content Standards for Teaching

One of the most important responsibilities of all health professionals is to teach the patient and his family what he must know to cope with the therapy he is receiving and to learn to prevent or cope with a health problem. There are two aspects to teaching: the content to be taught and the process of teaching. **Content standards** define the substance of what the patient needs to learn to prevent or cope with his health problem and therapy.

METHOD

The five steps in writing content standards for teaching a patient are:

1. Define the patient's health situation.
2. Identify the goals of teaching.
3. Develop the substance of teaching.
4. Combine the content standards in a logical order.
5. Establish the validity of the content standards.

When you have written content standards that meet the specifications described for each of these steps, you will have developed valid content standards that can be implemented.

STEP 1
Define the Patient's Health Situation

The description of the patient's health situation can assist you in defining pertinent goals. The description can be very brief but should be specific enough for you to identify the goals of teaching. For example, to say that a patient has incontinence is to describe a general health situation. The substance of teaching needed by the patient experiencing incontinence will vary depending on the type of incontinence.

On the other hand, the same content standards may be appropriate for several patients' health situations. The content standards for teaching a patient with chronic inefficient airway clearance are appropriate for patients experiencing emphysema, chronic bronchitis, and chronic asthma. To illustrate the steps in writing standards for teaching patients, the following health situation will be used as an example: *Adult Patient Experiencing Chronic Inefficient Airway Clearance*.[1] After you have defined the patient's health situation, go on to the next step.

STEP 2
Identify the Goals of Teaching

Read the description of the patient's health situation and identify the goals for the teaching required in the situation. A **goal** is an explicit statement describing what you plan to accomplish with your teaching.

After thinking about the description of the patient's health situation, ask yourself:

- What does the patient and family need to know to prevent or cope with a health problem?

For our example, *Adult Patient Experiencing Chronic Inefficient Airway Clearance*, the goals are:

- The patient will explain how his breathing is affected by chronic, inefficient airway clearance.
- The patient will modify his lifestyle as required.
- The patient will be able to list the community, state, and federal agencies that can be assistive to him and how to obtain needed services.
- The patient will be able to explain how to prevent infection.
- The patient will explain how to take his medications.
- The patient will demonstrate measures for effective airway clearance.

- The patient can explain how to identify environmental pollutants.
- The patient can explain how to modify his schedule for balancing rest and activity.
- The family, within its ability, will provide the support needed by the patient.

Note: When the goals are individualized for a specific patient, the exact date for the achievement of the goals must be defined.

STEP 3
Develop the Substance of Teaching

Now you are ready to identify the substance of the teaching required by the patient. To assist in the identification of the content, read each goal and ask yourself:

- What do I need to teach the patient to meet this goal?

In our example, the content standards for the goal *the patient will explain how his breathing is affected by a chronic inefficient airway clearance* are:

- Normal breathing
- Physiological changes in chronic inefficient airway clearance
- Factors that affect breathing

For the goal *the patient will modify his lifestyle as required,* the content standards are:

- Stopping smoking
- Use of oxygen, if needed
- Special diet, if needed
- Modification of job, if needed
- Decreased or different family responsibilities/tasks, as required
- Determination of financial situation

Now select another goal to identify the substance of teaching. The content standards for the goal *the patient will be able to list the community, state, and federal agencies that can be assistive to him, and how to obtain needed services* are:

- Examples of community agencies:
  Local American Lung Association, American Cancer Society, Visiting Nurses Association, hospice

- Examples of state and national agencies:
  Asthma and Allergy Foundation, Asthma Care Association of America, Lung Disease Hotline, National Institute of Allergies and Infectious Diseases, National Jewish Center for Immunology and Respiratory Medicine, National Heart, Lung and Blood Institute

For the goal *the patient will be able to explain how to prevent infection*, the content standards are:

- Increase fluid intake daily (unless contraindicated).
- Avoid crowds, especially during seasons when respiratory infections are common.
- Avoid contact with individuals having respiratory infections.
- Obtain flu and pneumonia vaccine at recommended intervals.
- Maintain optimal nutrition.
- Obtain adequate rest.
- Avoid stressors when possible.
- Avoid air pollution when possible.
- Identify early indicators of infection:
    a. Change in the color, odor, amount, and consistency of sputum
    b. Increased body temperature
    c. Increased shortness of breath

The content standards for the goal *the patient will explain how to take his medications* are:

- Action of the drugs
- When to take the medications
- How and when to alter dosage
- Side effects

For the goal *the patient will demonstrate measures for effective airway clearance,* the content standards are:

- Postural drainage
- Deep breathing techniques
- Coughing techniques
- Chest percussion
- Respiratory therapy
- Adequate hydration:
    a. Increased fluid intake

    b. Inhaled moisture

    c. Avoidance of caffeine or other diuretics

The content standards for the goal *the patient can explain how to identify environmental pollutants* are:

- Instruct him to avoid environmental pollutants such as tobacco smoke, aerosols, dust, and fumes.
- Provide written resources (when appropriate) such as the booklets "Dust Diseases Facts" and "Hints for Control of the Home Environment."

For the goal *the patient can explain how to modify his schedule for balancing rest and activity,* the content standards are based on the assessment of the patient's ability to do Activities of Daily Living, the amount and type of exercise and the schedule of rest periods will depend on the patient's exercise tolerance of the activities in his lifestyle.

The content standards for the goal *the family, within its ability, will provide the support needed by the patient* are:

- Patient's health problem
- Patient's treatment/care and assistance needed by the patient
- Factors affecting the patient's ability to do:
  - a. Activities of Daily Living
  - b. Roles within the family
  - c. Work
- Maintenance or improvement of relationships
- Support for changes in family members' roles due to patient's needs

As you read the content standards for these goals, notice that the methods of teaching the patient have not been included. Because many different methods of teaching can be used in implementing these content standards, process standards need to be developed for the most effective teaching methods.

After you have identified all the content standards, you are ready to proceed to the next step.

STEP 4
Combine the Content Standards in a Logical Order

Now review all the standards to ascertain whether you have identified all the content standards essential in teaching the patient regarding his health situation.

After doing this, combine the standards in a way that is most useful to the nurses who will be implementing them. Some content standards for teaching should be listed in chronological order. Certain standards, because they are implemented together, should be grouped together. Other content standards for teaching should be integrated into the intervention or unit of care that is related. The nurse will teach the patient while implementing the process standards for the intervention or unit of care. For example, the patient requiring perineal care post partum will also be taught how to do this care herself, after successfully demonstrating how to do it.

As you read the standards, think about how you would combine them. The following pattern is just one of the ways these content standards could be combined. The completed example lists the health situation, the goals of the teaching, and the content standards.

Unit of Care

Health Problem: Adult Patient Experiencing Chronic Inefficient Airway Clearance

Goals

1. The patient will explain how his breathing is affected by chronic inefficient airway clearance.
2. The patient will modify his lifestyle as required.
3. The patient will be able to list the community, state, and federal agencies that can be assistive to him and how to obtain needed services.
4. The patient will be able to explain how to prevent infection.
5. The patient will explain how to take his medications.
6. The patient will demonstrate measures for effective airway clearance.
7. The patient can explain how to identify environmental pollutants.
8. The patient can explain how to modify his schedule for balancing rest and activity.
9. The family, within its ability, will provide the support needed by the patient.

Note: When the goals are individualized for a specific patient, the exact date for the achievement of the goals must be defined.

Content Standards

Teach the patient and family:

1. Normal breathing
2. Physiological changes in inefficient airway clearance
3. Factors that affect breathing
4. Modification of his lifestyle
   a. Stopping smoking
   b. Use of oxygen, if needed
   c. Special diet, if needed
   d. Modification of job, if needed
   e. Decreased or different family responsibilities/tasks, as required
   f. Determination of financial situation
5. Community, state, and federal agencies: Local American Lung Association, American Cancer Society, Visiting Nurses Association, hospice, Asthma and Allergy Foundation, Asthma Care Association of America, Lung Disease Hotline, National Institute of Allergies and Infectious Diseases, National Jewish Center for Immunology and Respiratory Medicine, National Heart, Lung and Blood Institute
6. Measures to prevent infection:
   a. Increase fluid intake daily (unless contraindicated).
   b. Avoid crowds, especially during seasons when respiratory infections are common.
   c. Avoid contact with individuals having respiratory infections.
   d. Obtain flu and pneumonia vaccine at recommended intervals.
7. Maintain optimal nutrition
8. Obtain adequate rest
9. Avoid stressors when possible.
10. Avoid air pollution when possible.
11. Identify early indicators of infection:
    a. Change in the color, odor, amount, and consistency of sputum
    b. Increased body temperature
    c. Increased shortness of breath
12. Medication information
    a. Action of the drugs
    b. When to take the medications

      c. How and when to alter dosage

      d. Side effects

13. Measures for effective airway clearance:

      a. Postural drainage

      b. Deep breathing techniques

      c. Coughing techniques

      d. Chest percussion

      e. Respiratory therapy

      f. Adequate hydration

         1. Increased fluid intake

         2. Inhaled moisture

         3. Avoidance of caffeine or other diuretics

14. Identification of environmental pollutants

15. Avoidance of environmental pollutants such as tobacco smoke, aerosols, dust, and fumes

16. Provision of written resources (when appropriate) such as the booklets "Dust Diseases Facts" and "Hints for Control of the Home Environment"

17. Balancing rest and activity

18. Amount and type of exercise based on the assessment of the patient's ability to do Activities of Daily Living. (The amount and type of exercise and the schedule of rest periods will depend on the patient's exercise tolerance of the activities in his lifestyle.)

19. Factors affecting the support needed by the patient

      a. Patient's health problem

      b. Patient's treatment/care and assistance needed by the patient

      c. Factors affecting the patient's ability to do:

         1. Activities of Daily Living

         2. Roles within the family

         3. Work

20. Maintenance or improvement of relationships

21. Support for changes in family members' roles due to patient's needs

STEP 5
Establish the Validity of the Content Standards

Although you have developed content standards, these standards are not necessarily valid. Develop the outcome standards for teaching patients. You may want to read "Writing Outcome Standards" in chapter 3. Then refer to chapter 5 to establish the validity of the standards you have written.

After you have finished step 5, you have completed this section. You now need to decide what you want to read next. If you have not already done so, you may want to develop outcome standards related to the content standards you have written. If so, refer to chapter 3.

SECTION 3
Writing Content Standards for Therapeutic Communication

A **therapeutic communication** contains the content related to verbal intervention in a patient's sociologic or psychologic health problem or patient care need. A therapeutic communication can be a procedure or a unit of care. The **content standards** define the principles that should be included when intervening in a health problem or patient care need.

Because the effectiveness of therapeutic communication depends to a great extent on the nurses' unique use of self in communicating with the patient, the specific words and behavior important in the communication are not included in the standards. When a therapeutic communication is designed, outcome standards need to be written for the procedure or the unit of care.

METHOD

The five steps in developing content standards for therapeutic communication with patients are:

1. Define the procedure or unit of care.
2. Identify the goals of the communication.
3. Define the content of the therapeutic communication.
4. Combine the standards in a logical order.
5. Establish the validity of the content standards.

STEP 1
Define the Intervention or Unit of Care

Therapeutic communication can be implemented as a procedure or a unit of care. A **unit of care** can be titled as a nursing diagnosis, health problem, or patient care need. A **nursing diagnosis** is a clinical judgment about individual, family, or community responses to actual or potential health problems/ life processes. A **health problem** or **patient care need** can be defined as a collection of signs and symptoms that, taken together, constitute a picture of ill health or health care required by the patient. The patient care need or problem is expressed in a word/phrase that triggers in the mind of the clinician a picture of the health problem or patient care need and the interventions pertinent to its resolution. The example unit of care is *Altered Sensory Perception Related to Auditory Hallucinations.*

An operational definition of the unit of care is usually required to identify the goals of the nursing care. The definition must be meaningful to nurses implementing the standards as well as those writing the standards. An operational definition for auditory hallucinations is *the patient experiencing auditory hallucinations hears voices that he believes to be real and that others in the patient's environment can't hear.*

STEP 2
Identify the Goals of the Communication

For any communication with patients to be therapeutic, it must be goal-directed. Otherwise, the communication can become misdirected or useless to the patient. A **goal** is an explicit statement describing exactly what you plan to accomplish with the care. Goals should describe the expected patient outcomes. As you think about the reasons for implementing this intervention, ask yourself:

- What can therapeutic communication do to help the patient who is experiencing this nursing diagnosis, health problem, or patient care need?

The goals related to the unit of care *Altered Sensory Perception Related to Auditory Hallucinations* are:

- The patient will realize that the voices he hears are not heard by others.
- The patient will realize that taking medication has a direct connection with reducing the number of hallucinations.
- The patient will inform staff when hallucinations are occurring.

- The patient will remain focused on the current conversation and not respond to the hallucination for _____ minutes per day. (As the patient responds to the therapy, the number of minutes in the goal will increase.)
- The patient will complete a simple task such as _____ on a daily basis.
- The patient will work with family/staff and/or significant other(s) to identify the stressor(s) that may increase the frequency of hallucinations.
- The patient will not harm himself.

Note: When the goals are individualized for a specific patient, the exact date for the achievement of the goal must be defined.

STEP 3
Define the Content of the Therapeutic Communication

The content standards contain the principles of the *approach* to the patient so that all nurses implement these principles in all their interactions with the patient to provide a consistent approach. For each goal, ask yourself:

What must I do when communicating with this patient to meet this goal?

- Observe patients for verbal and nonverbal behavior related to hallucinations. (This behavior should be documented and communicated to others caring for the patient.)
- Explain to the patient that the "command voices" occur usually when he is experiencing increased anxiety and that these voices are not heard by others.
- Redirect the patient's attention to a specific activity. (This activity was defined during mutual goal setting between the nurse and the patient.)
- Avoid touching the patient without telling him you are going to touch him.
- Do not reinforce the hallucinations by agreeing with the patient. Assist the patient, when possible, to clarify reality.
- Encourage the patient to discuss the hallucinations with you.
- When the patient is not hallucinating:
    a. Assist him to identify stressors.
    b. Explain that the therapy he is receiving will decrease the number of hallucinations.

- Intervene as necessary when patient expresses ideas from the "command voices" that might cause the patient to harm himself. (This is a process standard.)

When you have identified all the principles of therapeutic communication related to this unit of care, you have developed content standards. Now, proceed to step 4.

STEP 4
Combine the Standards in a Logical Order

The completed unit of care lists the title and the goals and combines the content standards in the order of their use. The following order is just one approach to ordering content standards for this unit of care. Review this list of content standards and then order them in a way that is most useful to the nurses who will be implementing the standards.

Unit of Care

Altered Sensory Perception Related to Auditory Hallucination

Goals

1. The patient will not harm himself.
2. The patient will identify that the voices he hears are not heard by others.
3. The patient will realize that taking medication has a direct connection with reducing the number of hallucinations.
4. The patient will inform staff when hallucinations are occurring.
5. The patient will remain focused on the current conversation and not respond to the hallucination for _____ minutes per day. (As the patient responds to the therapy, the number of minutes in the goal will increase.)
6. The patient will complete a simple task such as _____ on a daily basis.
7. The patient will work with family/staff and/or significant other(s) to identify the stressor(s) that may increase the frequency of hallucinations.

Note: When the goals are individualized for a specific patient, the exact date for the achievement of the goals must be defined.

Content Standards

1. Observe patients for verbal and nonverbal behavior related to hallucinations. (This behavior should be documented and communicated to others caring for the patient.)
2. Explain to the patient that the "command voices" occur usually when he is experiencing increased anxiety and that these voices are not heard by others.
3. Redirect the patient's attention to a specific activity. (This activity was defined during mutual goal setting between the nurse and the patient.)
4. Avoid touching the patient without telling him you are going to touch him.
5. Do not reinforce the hallucinations by agreeing with the patient. Assist the patient, when possible, to clarify reality.
6. Encourage the patient to discuss the hallucinations with you.
7. When the patient is not hallucinating:
   a. Assist him to identify stressors.
   b. Explain that the therapy he is receiving will decrease the number of hallucinations.
8. Intervene as necessary when patient expresses ideas from the "command voices" that might cause the patient to harm himself.[3]

STEP 5
Establish the Validity of the Content Standards

Although you have developed content standards, these standards are not necessarily valid. Refer to chapter 5 to establish the validity of the standards.

Develop outcome standards for the outcomes of the therapeutic interaction. You may want to read "Writing Outcome Standards for Units of Care" in chapter 3.

SECTION 4

Writing Content Standards for Decision Making in Emergency Situations

Content standards need to be developed for decisions that are vital to the provision of nursing care. The importance of writing standards for nurses' decisions can be illustrated by the following example. There are three nurses working on a thirty-bed unit in a general hospital. A patient has a myocardial infarction. Only one of the three nurses knows what to do in this emergency. The explanation given by the other two nurses for why they do not know what to do is that there has not been such a emergency in that clinical unit for more than 3 years. The nurse who knows what to do is a nurse who frequently reviews his knowledge of care of patients during emergency situations. Thus, a patient might die if one of the nurses does not know what to do during the emergency.

Nurses are responsible for making appropriate decisions concerning the welfare of patients regardless of the frequency of occurrence of an emergency situation. If content standards are written for decisions nurses make in emergencies, nurses can review the standards frequently enough to retain their expertise when faced with an emergency.

Moreover, when content standards are developed for emergencies, better procedures and policies regarding the use of emergency equipment can be developed. For example, in a locked psychiatric unit, the door to the fire equipment cabinet was also locked. When asked what he would do in the event of a fire in the unit, each nurse said he would get the fire extinguisher. The nurse was then requested to get the equipment and bring it to the nurses' station, the simulated site of the fire. Each staff member went to the fire extinguisher cabinet and found it locked. Each said the cabinet was locked but did not know the location of the key. In this instance, because the fire equipment was used infrequently, the key had been lost. Thus, this equipment could not have been used when needed in a real fire. If content standards are written and reviewed frequently, nursing personnel will know how to function effectively in an emergency when it arises.

Content standards need to be written for decisions nurses make during emergencies. There are two components of these types of content standards: a description of the situation requiring a nurse's decision and the course of action for dealing with it.

METHOD

The method for writing content standards for emergencies involves three steps:

1. Describe the emergency.
2. Identify the appropriate course of action.
3. Establish the validity of the content standards.

Now study the description of each step.

STEP 1
Describe the Decision-making Situation

To identify those emergencies situations for which content standards need to be developed, ask yourself the following question:

• What emergencies confront nurses?

There are three types of emergencies that require nurses to intervene. The first type is a complication experienced by the patient. Some examples are cardiac arrest, attempted suicide, placenta previa, shock, airway obstruction, hemorrhage, and autonomic dysreflexia. Another type of emergency that affects groups of patients are natural disasters such as fire, flood, earthquake, tornado, hurricane, or blizzard.

Nurses also modify a procedure or discontinue the procedure when the patient may be experiencing an untoward effect of an intervention. Two examples of this type of situation are:

• The patient experiences pain during an enema.
• The patient's chest tube disconnects from the drainage system.

After you have identified an emergency, write a brief description of it.
In our example, a patient is experiencing *Pulmonary Edema*:

• Respiratory distress: labored, noisy breathing; frothy coughing, blood-tinged sputum; orthopnea; shortness of breath
• Restlessness, anxiety, confusion
• Fear of suffocation and dying
• Profuse perspiration

STEP 2
Identify the Course of Action Appropriate to the Situation

You need to think of the impact of the situation on the patient or the patient's family. As you do this, ask yourself:

- What should I do in this situation that will benefit the patient and the patient's family?

The possible courses of action might be to intervene yourself, to request intervention or assistance of someone with more expertise in dealing with the situation, or a combination of direct intervention and a request for assistance. In our example situation, a patient is experiencing *Pulmonary Edema*.

1. Position the patient in high Fowlers' position with lower limbs dependent. Provide support for the patient's arms.
2. Remain with the patient. Implement measures to decrease venous return and pulmonary congestion.
3. Provide emotional support.
4. Check vital signs every 15 minutes until stable, then 30 minutes for 3 hours. If stable, check vital signs every hour for 24 hours.
5. Observe for arrhythmias, hypoxia, hypercapnia, confusion, and stupor.

After you have identified all the content standards appropriate to the situation, proceed to the next step.

STEP 3
Establish the Validity of the Content Standards

Although you have developed content standards, they are not necessarily valid. Develop the outcome standards concerning the outcomes of the decision-making situation. You may want to review "Writing Outcome Standards" in chapter 3. Then refer to chapter 7 to establish the validity of the standards. You have completed this section.

SECTION 5

Writing Content Standards for Documentation

Content standards define what needs to be documented concerning the interventions being implemented, the patient's responses to the interventions and therapy, and the patient's progress toward the goals of the plan of care. The most important reason for documentation is to communicate to nurses and other health care professionals vital information needed to provide high-quality care to patients. Another essential reason for the documentation of the care is to meet legal and accrediting requirements. In many malpractice lawsuits, the lack of accurate documentation has incriminated health professionals. Agencies that accredit quality improvement programs have criteria related to documentation. Therefore, the content standards for documentation must meet the current legal and accrediting requirements.

Content standards are written to provide nurses with clear guidelines of what to record, yet permit them to individualize the data concerning each patient. Content standards should be developed for the documentation related to the process, content, and outcome standards for every nursing intervention and unit of care.

METHOD

The method for developing content standards for documentation contains the following five steps:

1. Collect the information essential to write the content standards.
2. Identify the data regarding the implementation of nursing care that must be recorded.
3. Identify the data concerning the effectiveness of nursing care that must be recorded.
4. Review the legal and accrediting requirements regarding the documentation of nursing care.
5. Combine the content standards in a logical order.
6. Establish the validity of the standards.

Now that you have read the method, study each step of the method, beginning with step 1.

STEP 1
Collect the Information Essential
to Write the Content Standards

Before you can identify the data that should be documented, you need to review the process, content, and outcome standards for a nursing intervention or the unit of care. These standards define:

a. Care provided to the patient and possible complications to avoid
b. Expected patient responses to the care
c. Expected outcomes of the care

In the example unit of care *Chronic Seizures in Children,* the *process standards* are:

1. Assign child to room near nurses station for close observation.
2. Apply a monitor to all infants and any child with a history of apnea or cyanosis during seizure episode.
3. Assess vital signs q4h.
4. Keep oxygen and suction set-up at the bedside at all times.
5. Observe events that lead up to seizures:
   a. Emotional outburst
   b. Noise or excitement
   c. Flashing or bright lights*
   d. Smells*
   e. Ringing in the ears*
6. Observe post-seizure behavior.
7. Administer anticonvulsants. Note their effect on the seizure pattern as well as the behavior of the child, and note side effects.

*If the child is old enough to describe events.

The *content standards* for teaching the parents during the seizure are:

1. Remain with the child.
2. Remove potentially harmful objects close to the child.
3. Do not restrain the child.
4. Do not open mouth or attempt to place anything in the mouth.
5. If necessary, suction nose and mouth of secretions.

6. Observe during the seizure:
   a. Onset
   b. Respiratory effort
   c. Behavior in chronological order
   d. Duration

The *outcome standards* at all times are:

1. The child remains free from injury during a seizure.
2. All seizures are accurately documented.
3. The child's parents can explain:
   a. What to do during a seizure
   b. What needs to be reported to nurses and the physician about the child's seizures
   c. The child's reponse to the therapy[4]

When you have identified all the process, content, and outcome standards for a nursing intervention or unit of care, proceed to step 2.

STEP 2
Identify the Data Regarding the Implementation of Nursing Care that Must Be Recorded

Some of the process standards of an intervention and unit of care must be documented. For example, if you are applying heat or cold to the patient's body, the length of application and the frequency of application need to be recorded. Other interventions require that observations made during the intervention be recorded. An example of this type of intervention is *Changing a Dressing*.

Now review the standards and think about the interventions and observations that need to be recorded. Ask yourself:

• What data need to be recorded to document the implementation of nursing care?
   a. Apply the monitor to all infants and any child with a history of apnea or cyanosis during seizure episode.
   b. Administer anticonvulsants. Note their effect on the seizure pattern as well as the behavior of the child and side effects.
   c. During and after the seizure, suction secretions of the child's nose and mouth when necessary.

Interventions and observations taught to parents post-seizure.

What data need to be documented to identify the patient's response to the therapy and nursing care?

- Vital signs q4h.
- Events that led to the seizure (if observed):
  a. Emotional outburst
  b. Noise or excitement
  c. Flashing or bright lights
  d. Smells
  e. Ringing in the ears
- During the seizure
  a. Onset
  b. Respiratory
  c. Behavior in chronological order
  d. Duration
- Post-seizure behavior
- Child's response to the therapy
- Parents' response to interventions and observations taught to them

After completing this task, proceed to step 3.

STEP 3
Identify the Data Concerning the Effectiveness of Nursing Care That Should Be Recorded

The patient's response to therapy and progress toward the goals of care are essential items to record. These outcomes will assist other health professionals in identifying what interventions should be implemented next in the patient's care.

Ask yourself:

What should be documented concerning the effectiveness of nursing care?

- The child remains free from injury during a seizure.
- All seizures are accurately documented.
- The child's parents can explain:
  a. What to do during a seizure
  b. What needs to be reported to nurses and the physician about the child's seizures
  c. Child's reponse to the therapy

The content of the observations overlaps the content of the outcome standards because the observations and the outcomes describe the patient's response to nursing care.

STEP 4
Review the Legal and Accrediting Requirements Regarding the Documentation of Nursing Care

After you have identified all the data that must be recorded to provide for the continuity and comprehensiveness of nursing care, review the current legal and accrediting requirements concerning documentation. Then write additional content standards as necessary or format the content standards that you have written to meet these requirements. For example, if you did not include the outcome standard *the child remains free from injury during a seizure* as a content standard, it should be added at this time. After completing this step, proceed to step 5.

STEP 5
Combine the Content Standards in a Logical Order

Now review all the standards to ascertain whether you have identified all the content standards. After doing this, combine the standards in a way that is most useful to the nurses who will be implementing them.

Unit of Care

Chronic Seizures in Children

Content Standards for Documentation

1. A monitor was applied to all infants and any child with a history of apnea or cyanosis during a seizure episode.
2. Vital signs were taken q4h.
3. Events that led to the seizure:
   a. Emotional outburst
   b. Noise or excitement
   c. Flashing or bright lights*
   d. Smells*
   e. Ringing in the ears*

*If the child is old enough to describe events.

4. During the seizure, record:
   a. Onset
   b. Respiratory effort
   c. Behavior in chronological order
   d. Duration
   e. Any suctioning of nose and mouth to remove secretions
   f. Any injuries
5. Post-seizure behavior
6. Child's response to the therapy
7. Parents' response to interventions and observations taught to them

Then proceed to step 6.

STEP 6
Establish the Validity of the Standards

The content standards you have written need to be reviewed by three nurses knowledgeable about the nursing care contained in the intervention or unit of care. This step is done to ensure the content validity of the standards. After the experts agree that these are the content standards for documentation for a specific nursing intervention or unit of care, the standards are valid.

SECTION 6
Writing Content Standards for Reporting

To provide for more rapid communication among health professionals and between less-prepared personnel and health professionals responsible for the patient's care, content standards are developed for the data that must be shared concerning the patient's responses to care and the patient's progress. Because the substance of the standards is the information required by other health professionals, you need to ask these professionals what data they require for making decisions.

In health agencies where less-prepared staff make observations while giving care instead of the registered nurse responsible for the patient, staff must know what needs to be reported to the registered nurse. These observations can be written on the plan of care used by the staff.

Content standards define what needs to be reported, to whom, and when. Some of the types of data that must be reported are the same as the data required to be documented. The major difference between the two types of content standards is that some data must be communicated more rapidly than is possible if the data are only recorded. This is necessary when another nurse or health professional must intervene immediately in the patient's health situation to prevent complications or to change the plan of care as a result of changes in the patient's condition. Content standards are developed for nursing interventions and units of care.

METHOD

The method for developing content standards for the recording of data contains the following five steps:

1. Determine the data that must be reported.
2. Decide to whom the data must be reported.
3. Specify when the data must be reported.
4. Combine the standards in a logical order.
5. Establish the validity of the standards.

STEP 1
Determine the Data That Must Be Reported

In order to identify situations requiring the reporting of data, you must first collect the information essential to the task. If you have developed the process and outcome standards for an intervention or unit of care, these standards and the goals of the care should be used to identify the data that must be reported. Then ask health professionals who need the information what specifics they require for decision making and intervention. A patient with a cast requires the following observations related to the interventions and outcomes of care:

- Observe the skin around the cast for :
  a. Color changes
  b. Edema
  c. Temperature
  d. Irritation

- Observe for changes in the pulses distal to the cast—compare one extremity to another.
- Observe for changes in sensation—decreased or numbness and tingling.
- Observe for sudden increases or decreases in the amount of pain.
- Observe for a decrease in movement of unaffected muscles.
- Observe for capillary refill (increased time for refill) distal to the cast—compare one extremity to another.
- Observe the cast for:
    a. Bleeding
    b. Indentations and cracks, if there are resulting pressure symptoms or impaired integrity of the cast
    c. Odor or drainage

After you have collected the necessary information, review it and ask yourself:

- What patient responses require the intervention of another health professional?

The following patient responses need to be reported:

- Skin around the cast for :
    a. Color changes
    b. Edema
- Changes in the pulses distal to the cast—compare one extremity to another
- Changes in sensation—decreased or numbness and tingling
- Sudden increases or decreases in the amount of pain
- Decrease in movement of unaffected muscles
- Capillary refill—increased time for refill
- Cast:
    a. Bleeding
    b. Indentations, if there are resulting pressure symptoms or softness
    c. Odor or drainage

After you have identified the patient responses that need to be reported, proceed to step 2.

STEP 2
Decide to Whom the Data Must Be Reported

Another important consideration in writing these content standards is the health professional to whom the data should be reported. After you have identified what data need to be reported, ask yourself:

- To whom should this data be reported?

In our example of the patient with a cast, the following data should be reported to the physician because it is the physician's responsibility to intervene if the patient experiences:

- Active bleeding in the wound
- Changes in motor function, sensory function
- Impaired circulation in the affected limb

Thus, observations that indicate any of these complications should be reported to the physician.

If there are nursing personnel observing the patient, all changes in the patient's status should be reported to the nurse responsible for the care of the patient. In addition to the data the nurse should report to the physician, the observation *irritation of the skin from the cast* should be reported to the nurse for intervention. Now proceed to the next step.

STEP 3
Specify When the Data Must Be Reported

The last component of the content standards is when the data must be reported. The time frame for reporting reflects what type of intervention is required or when the health professional needs this information to adjust the plan of care to prevent negative outcomes for the patient. To identify the "when" of the standards, review the "what" and the "to whom," and ask yourself:

- When must this data be reported?

In the example, the data that indicate the patient is experiencing imminent decreased motor function, sensory function, active bleeding, or circulatory impairment in the affected limb should be reported *immediately* to the physician. There are other observations, such as:

- Bleeding, if it is not extensive in a new cast
- Indentations/cracks in the cast or softness of the cast

Such observations need to be reported to the physician during patient rounds *as long as the patient is not experiencing symptoms requiring immediate attention.*

STEP 4
Combine the Standards in a Logical Order

Now review all the standards to ascertain whether you have identified all the content standards for reporting data related to this nursing intervention. Then combine the standards in a way that is most useful to the nurses implementing them.

The completed material identifies the unit of care and lists the content standards.

Unit of Care

Nursing Care of the Patient with a Cast

Content Standards

1. Report active bleeding in the wound, changes in motor function, sensory function, or impaired circulation in the affected limb immediately to the physician.
2. Report irritation of the skin from the cast to the registered nurse responsible for the patient (in addition to the symptoms that will be reported to the physician).

STEP 5
Establish the Validity of the Standards

The content standards need to be reviewed by three people knowledgeable about the nursing care related to the intervention or unit of care. This is done to establish the validity of the standards. After completing step 5, you will have completed this section.

NOTES

1. Carpenito, Lynda Juall. *Nursing diagnosis: Application to clinical practice* (4th ed.), p. 676. New York: J.B. Lippincott and Co., 1992.

2. Donna Cericola and the staff at Shore Memorial Hospital, Somers Point, N.J., 1992.

3. Staff nurses at the Delaware State Hospital, Wilmington, Del., 1992.

4. Dianne Charsha, clinical specialist at Shore Memorial Hospital, Somers Point, N.J., 1993.

6

The Meaningful Standard: Editing for Precision in Meaning

A meaningful standard is like a sharp-focus photograph. Those who look at the photograph perceive the picture as clearly as the photographer saw through the lens. A meaningful process standard defines what must be done to achieve positive outcomes for patients receiving the procedure/unit of care. A meaningful outcome standard is a clear description of the health status of the patient/family after they have received care. You should approach the writing of a standard with the precision of an expert photographer, because a meaningful standard precludes any possible misunderstanding of its meaning.

Because a standard is a collection of words and symbols, word choice is especially important when writing a meaningful standard. You are searching for the group of words and symbols that will communicate your intent precisely.

The editorial changes you make are essential to establishing the validity of the standards. Therefore, you should follow the recommendations for editing the standards before you attempt to establish their validity.

SECTION 1
Word Choice

Some words are open to a wide range of interpretation. To the extent that you use these words, you leave yourself open to being misunderstood. The following are examples of words with multiple meanings.

Knows, understands   *Normal*
Frequently   *As possible*

Let's now consider each of these words and suggest revisions to clarify the meaning of each.

KNOWS OR *UNDERSTANDS*

When you see *knows* or *understands* in a standard, you might wonder how you can tell if the patient knows or understands. Consider, for example, the statement *the patient knows how to prevent an elevation in his blood pressure.* Until you define what the patient does when demonstrating that she knows or understands, the standard is not meaningful. Items that might be included in teaching the patient about her hypertension are:

- Factors that elevate and lower blood pressure
- How to increase potassium intake when taking certain diuretics
- How to identify sodium or vasoconstrictor medication in other medications
- How to establish a realistic schedule of rest and activity
- How to establish a regular exercise routine
- How to use relaxation techniques and imagery
- How to identify stresses and find ways to eliminate them
- How to identify signs and symptoms to report to the physician

The patient who knows or understands can demonstrate procedures that must be followed. For example, a standard could be written as follows: *The patient demonstrates how to take his blood presssure.* This demonstration would include:

- Correct application of the blood pressure cuff
- Correct location of the arterial pulse
- Proper inflation of the blood pressure cuff
- Accurate interpretation of the blood pressure reading

• Results that must be communicated to the physician

Even if you believe that all staff caring for the patient should know what is included in the patient's demonstration of taking a blood pressure, include this content in the standard. It is useful to have this type of information available in a place of easy access for new clinicians and students.

FREQUENTLY

In many standards, the word *frequently* is used to identify when an intervention or observation needs to be done. But how often is *frequently*? Every clinician knows what he means by frequently, but rarely do two clinicians have the same understanding of the time frame. You should eliminate *frequently* as a time designation and replace it with words having more specific meaning, such as *every 2 hours.*

NORMAL

Normal is a word that can have a clear meaning, but its use can result in ambiguity in the meaning of a standard. Consider the statement *the characteristics of the sputum are within normal limits.* The meaning of this use of *normal* is clear because it refers to the values that have been established and accepted for the characteristics of the sputum of a healthy individual.

On the other hand, suppose the word *normal* is used to refer to the patient's premorbid baseline characteristics. The meaning of the word when used in this way may be unclear because some of the premorbid characteristics of this patient may not be within psychological and physiological ranges established as normal. Therefore, you should use the word *normal* only when referring to those ranges of human behavior established as being consistent with optimum health.

AS POSSIBLE

The phrase *as possible* is highly ambiguous and commonly found in standards. When used in a standard, the items with *as possible* as a time frame are usually not done at all by a busy clinician. If a time dimension is required in a standard, when the standard needs to be done should be specified. *Every hour* is an unambiguous time dimension.

Besides the examples discussed above, many other words have multiple meanings. Examine each of your standards to ascertain whether you have included words or phrases that might be unclear to other clinicians.

TESTS FOR CLARITY OF MEANING

After you are sure that the standards are clearly written, ask at least five clinicians who will be implementing the standards what each standard means to them. Compare their explanations with what you intended when you wrote the standard. If the meaning of the standard is the same, the standard is meaningful.

Another test to ascertain whether a standard is meaningful is to observe clinicians performing a procedure or implementing a unit of care. Compare the clinicians' actions with the process standards you have written for that procedure/unit of care. The standards that match the clinicians' actions are written in a meaningful way.

If a process standard you have written does not correspond to the clinicians' actions, ask the clinicians if they are implementing the standards as they understand them. However, do not change the standard if the clinicians' actions are inconsistent with their understanding of the standards.

FORM OF THE STANDARD

The standard should be written in a manner that enables you to decide whether the standard has been met. Specifically, the standard should be clear enough that you can say "the standard was met" or "the standard was not met" when observing the implementation of a standard or the outcomes of care. The best way to achieve this clarity is to put only one standard in each process or outcome statement.

Clear Examples	*Unclear Examples*
Absence of diarrhea	Absence of diarrhea and excoriation of the perineal area
Gently insert the rectal tube three inches into the rectum.	Gently insert the rectal tube three inches into the rectum and raise the enema bag twelve to fourteen inches above the anus and allow the solution to run in slowly.

Suppose you were evaluating whether the first outcome statement of the unclear examples has been met. You observe the patient has no diarrhea but does have excoriation of the perineal area. It is impossible to determine whether this outcome standard has been met because two outcomes are combined in it. Now look at the first of the clear outcome statements. It is easy to ascertain whether this standard was met.

Now consider the second example. In the clear example only one intervention is listed, while in the unclear category, there are two. It is possible to (1) insert the rectal tube three inches into the rectum and not meet the standard (2) by holding the enema container too high. In summary, it is essential to write only one standard in each statement.

After you have reviewed all the standards you have written and revised them as necessary to clarify their meaning and form, you are ready to add any necessary qualifying statements.

SECTION 2
Qualifying Statements

Sometimes it is essential to add qualifying statements to standards to make them meaningful. A qualifying statement is a group of words that adds clarity to the meaning of the standard. For process standards a qualifying statement is added to make the standards appropriate to all patients requiring the procedure/unit of care. There are two types of qualifying statements appropriate for outcome standards:

a. Relates to the patient's individual characteristics and environment

b. Defines the clinician's responsibilities in relation to the outcomes of care

Now review the process and outcome standards you have written to identify if they need a qualifying statement.

QUALIFYING STATEMENTS: PROCESS STANDARDS

The condition and characteristics of the patient and patient's environment have an important effect on whether clinicians can meet the process standards they have developed. Qualifying statements can make the standards appropriate for the care of patients with different characteristics.

For each process standard, ask yourself:

- Can every patient receive the care described in this process standard and have a positive outcome?

If this answer is "yes," you do not need a qualifying statement. If the answer is "no," a qualifying statement should be included.

For example, a process standard for the unit of care *Care of the Immobilized Patient* is *Encourage fluids up to 3000 cc.* This standard is appropriate for all patients who are in fluid and electrolyte imbalance. You can add a qualifying statement to the standard that will make it appropriate to the care of all immobilized patients: *Encourage fluids up to 3000 cc, unless contraindicated.* This qualifying phrase cues the clinician to think about the other health problems/patient care needs before encouraging fluid for the patient. For patients with edema or increasing intracranial pressure, fluids may be restricted.

Some process standards cannot be met by patients with certain health problems. Consider the following process standards for the procedure *Gastrostomy Feedings: Assist the patient into high Fowler's position.* The qualifying phrase *unless contraindicated* is important to add to this process statement because some patients may be unable to assume the position that would be optimal for gastrostomy feedings. Other examples of items found in process standards that might be contraindicated are specific positions, amount of exercise/activity, and the amount of oral fluid ingested per day.

For each process standard involving patient participation, ask yourself:

- Can every patient receiving the care described in this process standard do what is written in this standard?

If this answer is "yes," you do not need a qualifying statement. If the answer is "no," a qualifying statement should be included.

In summary, qualifying statements must be written for some process standards to make them appropriate for all patients requiring them. When the same qualifying statement is needed for several standards in the same unit of care/procedure, an asterisk(*) is placed beside the standards and the qualifying statement is written as a footnote following the list of process standards.

QUALIFYING STATEMENTS: OUTCOME STANDARDS

The health status and characteristics of the patient have an important effect on whether an outcome standard is appropriate for evaluating a specific patient's care. Some patients cannot progress to an outcome standard that is defined as physiologically or psychologically normal. Qualifying statements can make the outcome standards appropriate for patients with chronic health problems or patients with altered anatomy and physiology from surgery or other therapies. The qualifying statement refers the clinician implementing the outcome standards to a description of the patient at a previous point in time.

For each outcome standard you have written, ask yourself:

- Would it be possible for all patients to achieve the outcome standard if the care is provided according to the process standards?

If the answer is "yes," you do not need a qualifying statement. If the answer is "no," a qualifying statement should be included.

Consider the following outcome standard for *Care of the patient with urinary incontinence:*

At all times there is an absence of inflammation or skin breakdown in the perineal area. If this finding was abnormal before admission, the finding is improved from the original observation after the patient has received care.

The qualifying statement in the second sentence is important because some patients may have had inflammation and/or skin breakdown in the perineal area on admission. This statement alerts the clinician implementing the outcome standards to check the patient's records if a negative outcome appears when the patient's care is evaluated.

Frequently, more than a single health professional contributes to the outcomes of care experienced by the patient. Thus, qualifying statements that define the clinician's responsibility for the outcomes need to be attached to many outcome statements. For example, one of the outcome standards related to the unit of care *Potential for Arrhythmias* is:

At all times the patient is not experiencing life-threatening arrhythmias. *If the patient's cardiac rhythm changes or she experiences the following symptoms, the physician was notified: dizziness, fainting, irregular pulse, palpitations, fainting, shortness of breath, fatigue, pallor, cyanosis, chest pain, or weakness.*

The responsibility of the clinician in this standard is to observe the patient and report any significant changes to the physician. The phrase in italics makes the standard more meaningful because it clarifies the clinician's responsibility.

To assist you in identifying whether this type of qualifying statement is needed for the standard you are developing, ask yourself:

- What is the clinician's responsibility in relation to achieving the outcome standard?

The answer to this question clarifies the clinician's responsibility, thus making the standard more meaningful to the clinicians implementing it.

The following example defines the clinicians' responsibility concerning an outcome standard for *Care of the Patient Receiving Antibiotics*.

The patient is not experiencing an allergic reaction to the medication. *If the patient experiences a skin rash, dermatitis, hives, pruritus, wheezing, or fever, the physician is notified immediately.*

In this example, the clinician cannot be totally responsible for preventing an allergic reaction in the patient resulting from the nature of the antibiotic therapy. Thus, the qualifying statement in italics has been added. It is the clinician's responsibility to observe the patient frequently for beginning signs and symptoms of an allergic reaction and report them; the physician has the responsibility to order therapy for the allergic reaction when it occurs.

In summary, qualifying statements must be written for some outcome standards to make them appropriate for patients with various characteristics and health problems and to define the clinician's responsibility. When the same qualifying statement is needed for several standards, an asterisk (*) is placed beside the standards and the qualifying statement is placed in a footnote following the list of outcome standards.

After you have made sure your standards have a precise meaning and have added any necessary qualifying statements, you are ready to establish the validity of the standards.

7

Establishing the Validity and Efficiency of Standards

This chapter contains the methods for establishing the validity and efficiency of the standards. All the process, content, and outcome standards you write must meet the requirements described in this chapter before they are implemented.

Validity refers to the degree to which evidence supports inferences made from test scores.[1] In a health care context, validity can be defined as the care provided to patients (implemented process and content standards) that consistently results in positive outcomes (outcome standards).

Efficiency is defined as acting effectively with a minimum of waste expense or unnecessary effort.[2] In a health care context, efficiency can be defined as the combination of interventions and observations in a procedure or unit of care that require the fewest resources and time to implement, yet result in positive outcomes for patients.

The validity of the standards must be established before the efficiency can be determined. The standards must be tested to ensure that patients are experiencing positive outcomes before identifying what resources are required to implement the standards. If you attempt to test the standards for efficiency before they are valid, patients might experience negative out-comes before the right combination of resources can be identified that will result in positive outcomes.

Section 1 of this chapter describes the method for establishing the validity of the standards. Section 2 presents the method for establishing the efficiency of the standards.

SECTION 1

Establishing the Validity of the Standards

Before undergoing the tests for validity, all standards must be edited for precision in meaning, as described in chapter 6. Then they are ready to be tested for validity. There are two types of validity that should be established: content and criteria-related (predictive) validity.

A standard is **valid** to the extent that it defines:

a. An intervention or observation that must be implemented

b. An outcome of care that can be expected to occur when the care provided meets a need or resolves a health problem for patients.

CONTENT VALIDITY

Content validity is defined as the degree to which a sample of items on a test is representative of the same domain of content.[3] The first step in establish-ing the content validity of the standards of care is to identify a minimum of three resources. These resources can be:

a. Clinicians knowledgeable about the care and expected outcomes

b. Written sources that define the interventions, observations, and out-comes of care

If you have selected clinicians, show the standards to them and ask the following questions.

For process and content standards:

• Do these standards describe the care related to this procedure/unit of care?

• Are any process or content standards missing?

For the outcome standards:

- Are these the outcomes expected if the care related to this procedure/ unit of care is administered effectively?
- Are any outcomes missing from this list?

If the clinicians agree that the process, content, and outcome standards are the correct answers to the questions, the text of the standards contains content validity.

Or, you can identify the answers to the above questions in the content of the most current written sources—textbooks, journal articles, and documents containing legal requirements.

The content standards for the reporting and recording of data require only content validity. After the other standards have passed the test for content validity, they are ready to be tested for criterion related validity.

CRITERION-RELATED (PREDICTIVE) VALIDITY

Another type of validity essential for all process and outcome standards and most content standards is a strong, positive relationship between the process, content, and the outcome standards. **Criterion-related (predictive) validity** demonstrates that test scores (standards that were implemented) are systematically related to one or more outcome criteria (outcome standards).[4]

The major reason for establishing this type of validity for standards you are developing is that, in the past, many standards of care have *not* been tested to ascertain whether positive outcomes result for the patient after care has been administered. The question to be answered during the testing of the standards is:

- When the interventions and observations are implemented, do positive outcomes result for the patient?

After testing has been completed, if a consistent positive relationship exists between the effective implementation of the process/content standards that result in positive outcomes for the patients, then the process/ content and outcome standards are valid and ready to be implemented.

Before beginning the testing process, you need to write all the process, content, and outcome standards for the procedure/unit of care that will be tested. After completing this task, you are ready to develop the data collection sheets needed for testing.

DATA COLLECTION TOOLS

Supply the information for all the categories on the Data Collection Tool (figure 7.1). First complete the data in the heading of the Data Collection Tool:

- Title: Insert the title of the procedure/unit of care.
- Goals: List the goals. If you find you can collect data for more than one goal at the same time, put the goals and associated standards on the same tool.
- Data source: Enter a number to identify the patient for data analysis.

Note: The patient(s) must remain anonymous and the data collected must be kept confidential.

- Date: Insert the date of the data collection.
- Location: Enter the location of the data collection (the patient's room/ bed number, patient's home, type of clinic)
- Standards: Insert the outcome standards related to the goals.

Title: Administration of an Enema

Goal: The patient will have a bowel movement.

Data source: 364253   Location: 4 South   Date: 4/4/93

Yes	No	Outcome Standards
		1. The patient had a bowel movement.
		2. The patient has decreased abdominal distention.

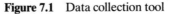

Figure 7.1   Data collection tool

List the standards in a logical order for data collection. The order may be chronological or the standards may be grouped according to which data can be collected together.

In summary, the Data Collection Tool should contain the following items:

- Title of the procedure/unit of care
- Goals of the procedure/unit of care
- Source of the data collection
- Date of the data collection
- Location of the data collection
- Columns for "yes" and "no" to the left of the process, content, or outcome standards

DATA COLLECTION

Now you are ready to begin the data collection process. There are two techniques for collecting data to establish the validity of the standards you have written. The first is to observe the clinician giving the care and then to collect data on the outcomes. The second method is to insist that the clinicians implement the care according to the written standards and then collect the data on the outcomes.

Regardless of which technique you use, be sure that the staffing is sufficient for clinicians to implement the standards fully. One reason clinicians do not implement standards is they cannot complete their assignments in one shift. In order to establish the validity of the standards, clinicians must implement the process standards fully. Thus, ensure adequate staffing on the clinical units used for establishing the validity of standards.

Before observing the clinician administering care, obtain the permission of the patient to observe, explaining why you want to do the observation. If the patient gives approval, observe the clinician administering the care and compare the clinician's performance with the process and/or content standards.

The second technique involves the clinician's cooperation. Review the process standards with those clinicians who will be participating. Emphasize the importance of implementing process standards; if the process standards are not met, you cannot establish the validity of the process or outcome standards. Although this technique is less expensive than the first because observers are not required, the technique is fraught with potential for error. The success of this technique depends on complete cooperation of the clinicians implementing the process standards.

Then, collect data on the outcomes. As soon as the outcomes of the care are apparent, observe them and mark the Data Collection Tool accordingly. For each testing of a set of standards, make ten observations of the process, content, and outcomes of care. The testing procedure should be repeated three times for each set of standards. After you have completed your observations, the Data Collection Tool will look similar to the one in figure 7.2.

There are some rules to follow during the testing to establish validity.

1. You need to collect data on the outcomes of care administered by *more than one* clinician. (It is essential to rule out the additional therapeutic effects of a particular clinician.)
2. The data collection should occur over several days to rule out the effect of the environment on the outcomes of care.
3. You should collect outcome data only on patients whose clinicians are implementing the process or outcomes standards you are testing.

DATA ANALYSIS

The initial step in data analysis is to total the number of "yes" and "no" checkmarks for each standard. Then apply the following decision rule to

---

Title: Administration of an Enema

Goal: The patient will have a bowel movement.

Data source: 364253   Location: 4 South   Date: 4/4/93

Yes	No	Outcome Standards
11111 11111		1. The patient had a bowel movement.
11111 11111		2. The patient has decreased abdominal distention.

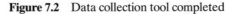

Figure 7.2   Data collection tool completed

each of the standards on the Data Collection Tool: Of the ten observations, if there are nine or ten marked in the "yes" column, the standard was met. If there are eight or fewer marks in the "yes" column, the standard was not met. (See figure 7.2.)

After you have identified which standards have been met, look at each goal on the Data Collection Tool and ask yourself:

- Have all of the process or content standards for this goal been met?

If the answer is "yes," then look at the outcome standards for the same goal and ask:

- Did positive outcomes result from the care that was administered to meet this goal?

If the process and content standards are met and positive outcomes result, a positive relationship results between the interventions implemented and positive outcomes for the patient.

Process or Content Standards Met→ Positive Outcomes

Although you can draw conclusions from one testing, it is better to retest the relationship between process or content and outcome standards two more times before drawing conclusions. If a positive relationship between the standards results in all tests, the process or content and outcome standards are valid.

What conclusion can you draw from the following diagram?

Process or Content Standards Met→ Negative Outcomes

When this occurs, it is obvious that the process standards are not valid. You are left with a puzzle to solve. You need to ask yourself:

- What additional interventions are required for the patient to experience positive outcomes?
- If the interventions are appropriate, do they need to be done more frequently or in a different sequence to achieve positive outcomes?

For example, suppose you change the position of an immobilized patient and assist him to deep breathe and cough every 2 hours, with the result that the patient is experiencing respiratory congestion. You may consider adding an additional intervention, such as increasing the patient's oral fluids, to the patient's plan of care. You can also approach this problem by thinking that the patient may need to be turned more frequently or receive a consultation from Respiratory Therapy. If you are at a loss about what to do, review the literature or ask resource people for assistance. After you decide which intervention/observations need to be changed, develop these standards, collect more data about them, and analyze the data. If the process or content standards are met and negative outcomes again result, continue to change one aspect of the care at a time until positive outcomes occur.

You can draw no conclusions from the following results:

Process or Content Standards Not Met→ Positive or Negative Outcomes

Clinicians must implement the process or content standards before the validity of the process or content standards and outcome standards can be established.

After you have finished establishing the validity of the standards, proceed to establish the efficiency of the standards in section 2.

SECTION 2
Improving the Efficiency of the Standards

Many procedures and units of care have been handed down for centuries from one generation of clinicians to another. Of these procedures and units of care, most have not been tested for their efficiency.

Efficiency is defined as "acting effectively with a minimum of wasted expense or unnecessary effort."[5] Efficiency in clinical terms can be defined as the combination of interventions and observations in each procedure and unit of care that requires the fewest resources and time to implement, yet results in positive outcomes for patients. After establishing their validity the standards define the text in the procedures and units of care that result in positive outcomes for patients. Because the cost of implementing the standards is vital in an era of limited resources and funding, you need to identify the combination of interventions and observations within each procedure and unit of care that requires the *fewest resources and shortest time* to implement yet *results in the same positive outcomes for patients*. In addition, increasing the efficiency of health care will provide more rest for patients; the patients may not need to be disturbed as frequently for their care. There are several ways to increase the efficiency of the standards:

1. Decreasing the frequency of implementing standards

2. Impact of equipment on the time required for care
3. Various combinations of interventions/observations

DECREASING THE FREQUENCY OF IMPLEMENTATION OF STANDARDS

As you review the procedures and units of care you are implementing, you need to ask yourself the following question:

• Can an intervention or observation be implemented fewer times a day and still result in the same positive outcomes for a patient?

For example, passive range of motion exercises usually are done four times every day to maintain the mobility of the patient's joints. It requires 5 minutes to assist the patient with these exercises. If doing the procedure once a day would result in the same positive outcomes, the patient would be able to rest those extra minutes and it would save 15 minutes of clinicians' time. While a savings of 15 minutes does not appear to be a large, if the clinician were caring for five patients requiring this procedure, it would save 75 minutes a day.

Now suppose it were possible to do the procedure 3 days a week instead of 7 days a week with the same positive outcomes. There would be additional time for the patient to rest and a greater savings of clinicians' time. And, if the exercises are done in the home, it would require fewer visits to the patient, thus saving travel time.

IMPACT OF EQUIPMENT ON THE TIME REQUIRED FOR CARE

Some procedures/units of care require equipment to implement the standards. There are products made by various companies to implement the same procedure. One of these products may require less time for clinicians to implement the standards than others. If the outcomes for the patient are as positive with use of the various products, the one saving clinicians' time should be selected. When testing equipment from various companies to determine which one will be purchased, you need to ask yourself the following question:

- Can the use of different equipment/supplies reduce the time it takes to do a specific procedure and still result in the same positive outcomes for a patient?

VARIOUS COMBINATIONS OF INTERVENTIONS/OBSERVATIONS

As clinicians implement a specific unit of care, they may identify other interventions that are more efficient. For example, when assisting a patient who has had abdominal surgery out of bed, if the patient is assisted to bend her knees and turn as a log when changing positions or getting out of bed, the patient is able to turn more easily and frequently requires less time to turn or transfer out of bed. This approach for moving a patient also causes less discomfort than other turning positions for patients after abdominal surgery.

As clinicians implement the standards, they should be asking themselves the following question:

- Can a different combination of interventions/observations be implemented and still result in the same positive outcomes for patients requiring this unit of care ?

TESTING THE EFFICIENCY OF THE STANDARDS

Efficiency can be defined as the combination of interventions and observations within each procedure and unit of care that require the fewest resources and time to implement, yet result in the same positive outcomes for patients. In studying the definition you will realize that the validity of the standards of the procedures and units of care must be established before you begin to establish the efficiency of the standards.

Before proceeding to improve the efficiency of any of the standards of care, you need to identify which standards of care require your attention first. The criteria for selection include:

- Those procedures and units of care that are implemented *very frequently.* Example: Administering intravenous medications and fluids
- Those interventions and observations that are *time-consuming.* Example: Obtaining pulmonary artery wedge pressure readings

Data Collection

When the standards of care are valid, develop the data collection tool containing the outcome standards as described in section 1 of this chapter. Then teach the clinician who will be implementing the standards the changes in the procedure/unit of care. The clinician implements the standards of care for one patient, while closely observing the patient's response to the care and the patient's progress toward the goals of care. If the patient's responses remain positive throughout the implementation of the changes, then implement the changes with a second patient. On the other hand, if the patient begins to experience a negative response, immediately increase the frequency of the interventions in the original standard of care.

The number of patients to be tested for each change and the data analysis are the same as for establishing the validity of the standards. As with establishing the validity of the standards, **the clinicians must implement the process and content standards before data related to patient outcomes can be gathered.**

SUMMARY

This chapter contains the method for establishing the validity and efficiency of the process, content, and outcome standards.

When the standards you have written have met the requirements for validity and efficiency specified in this chapter, they are ready to be implemented.

Now that you have finished this chapter, you may want to read chapter 8, "Implementing Standards."

NOTES

1. American Psychological Association. *Standards for educational and psychological testing*, p.9. Washington, D.C.: Author, 1985.
2. *The American heritage dictionary*, p.587. Boston, Mass.: Houghton Mifflin Co., 1992.
3. American Psychological Association, op. cit., p.10.
4. Ibid., p.11.
5. *The American heritage dictionary*, op. cit., p.9.

8

Implementing Standards of Care: Quality Management

After the standards you have developed have passed the tests for validity and efficiency, they are ready to be implemented. In addition to valid and efficient standards an organizational structure that facilitates clinicians' implementation of the standards and the commitment of administrators to the provision of continuous quality improvement is required in order for all patients to experience positive outcomes.

The JCAHO has identified common weaknesses in current practice that inhibit the provision of quality care in health care organizations:

1. A frequent focus only on the clinical aspects of care; for example, a focus on what the clinicians do with a patient rather than on the full series of interrelated governance, managerial, support, *and* clinical processes that affect patient outcomes

2. A frequent compartmentalization of QA activities in accordance with hospital structure rather than organizing quality improvement activities around the flow of patient care, in which the interrelated processes are often cross-disciplinary and cross-departmental.

3. A frequent focus on only the performance of individuals, especially on problem performance, rather than on how well the processes in which they participate are performed, how well the processes are coordinated and integrated, and how the processes can be improved

4. Frequently initiating action only when a problem is identified, rather than also trying to find better ways to carry out the processes

5. Separating appropriateness and effectiveness of care from the efficiency of care, rather than integrating efforts to improve patient outcomes with efforts to improve efficiency[1]

Failure to reach a desired level of performance usually relates to systems problems or to causes external to the system.[2] Deming, a pioneer in improving the quality of the outcomes of organizations, has stated that "85 percent of all errors are system errors, not employee errors."[3] His approach to quality is a systems approach designed to improve the effectiveness of operational service and reduce cost by concentrating the entire organization's efforts on processes that improve the quality of patient outcomes.[4] While standards define the quality of care that must be implemented by clinicians, the entire organization must focus on processes that result in positive outcomes for patients.

Where do you begin to imbed quality into the tapestry of the organization? Because everyone in the organization must work to achieve optimal quality, the overall mission statement that defines quality for the entire organization is a prime place to start. But first, how is quality in health care organizations being defined?

DEFINING QUALITY

There are many names for the definition of quality in health care organizations (quality management, quality improvement, continuous quality improvement). Let us look at some of the definitions of quality in the literature.

Katz and Green's definition of quality management is based on the premise that the quality within an organization is manageable, that it is within the scope of each individual within the organization to achieve quality as it relates to his/her job.[5]

Crosby defines quality management as a "systematic way of guaranteeing that organized activities happen the way they are planned."[6] He believes that the assumption of quality, meaning luxury or goodness, should be dispelled. What quality means is conformance to requirements.[7] It is the prevention of problems by "creating attitudes and controls" for preventing problems.[8]

Peters defines quality improvement "as the primary source of cost reduction."[9] All parts of the company must be part of the program. "Effective quality programs yield not only improved quality but lasting cost reductions as well."[10]

Dennis O'Leary, president of the Joint Commission on Accreditation of Health Services, has stated that "the pursuit of improvement in quality and efficiency in health care organizations is crucial to economic survival."[11] Masters and Schmele define total quality management as a "long term customer oriented cultural change."[12]

In summary, total quality management or continuous quality improvement is to "do the right thing right the first time, on time, all the time, and to strive always for improvement and customer satisfaction."[13]

While the names of the definitions are continually changing, there are two diverse assumptions inherent in the programs. One assumption is that "quality can be defined, managed, and problems that interfere with quality can be prevented."[14] The somewhat opposing definition is that "quality improvement is a never-ending journey."[15] These assumptions not only dictate how quality is defined but also guide the changes that are made in the structure of the organization to maintain or improve the quality of care.

In this chapter ideas related to quality management and quality improvement will be included. Compatible strategies of quality management will be presented. There are three sections in this chapter. Section 1 describes the importance of standards in an organization and the value of implanting them into the work of administrators and clinicians. The issues affecting evaluation of care, as well as the methodology for evaluation, are included in section 2. Section 3 contains the characteristics of the quality improvement team and its vital function in improving the quality of patient care.

SECTION 1
Embedding Standards into the Organization

The first step is to write a Mission Statement containing a definition of quality that is unambiguous and understood by all persons working in the organization. Then the administrators must communicate the Mission Statement to all persons in the organization. The commitment to quality as defined in the Mission Statement must be expressed in the way all employees and administrators do their work. Peters has stated, "A commitment to cost-effective quality is generated from the top down of a health care organization. It must permeate each level of the organization and be viewed as an integral part of each individual's responsibilities. Quality must be at the top of every agenda."[16] The structure and the policies must be reshaped to reflect the values and the commitment to make changes to achieve quality care. Every employee and every administrator must be involved in the effort to constantly improve work processes.[17] Every job must be analyzed to determine how that job reflects the values of the organization and the specifications of the job that must be met to contribute to the quality of the care provided.

Administrators must therefore design an effective organizational structure that will:

a. Facilitate the implementation of efficient as well as valid standards of care
b. Facilitate effective communication among the health professionals and departments
c. Encourage and reward cooperation among departments instead of rewarding stand-alone fiefdoms
d. Facilitate the rapid collection of data and data analysis related to patient outcomes throughout the organization
e. Spearhead organizational change as required to prevent negative patient outcomes
f. Develop reward systems for workers throughout the organization for quality in their performance

STANDARDS OPERATIONALIZE COMMITMENT TO QUALITY CARE

"The value system of the organization is made explicit by its written standards."[18] Meaningful standards provide the clear picture of organizational values. Written standards operationalize the commitment of quality. They define for the staff those interventions and patient outcomes for which they are held accountable.[19]

Crosby emphasizes "conformance to requirements; requirements that are clearly and specifically stated for each job."[20] All personnel must have a clear picture of how their responsibilities/actions relate to the total picture of providing quality. They must understand that if they don't fulfill their individual responsibilities, there will be a gap in the quality provided by the organization. For example:

- If staff do not follow the standards of care, or the administrative processes do not facilitate the implementation of the standards, the result will be negative patient outcomes. In addition, the organization may experience very costly legal problems.
- If staff and administrators do not implement the requirements of third-party payers and accrediting agencies, the organization will experience underreimbursement of costs incurred and/or upheaval due to a negative evaluation by the accrediting agencies.

Thus, all administrators, clinicians, and staff must operationalize the values of quality management every day in their work or:

1. Patients may not experience positive outcomes.
2. The organization can experience serious and sometime irreversible problems.

STANDARDS EMBEDDED INTO THE WORK OF CLINICIANS

After the standards you have developed have passed the tests for validity and efficiency, they are ready to be implemented. The standards must be integrated into all aspects of the work and decision making of clinicians in order to provide positive outcomes for patients. The valid and efficient process standards (interventions and observations), content standards, and outcome standards must be implemented during all aspects of patient care, from assessment through evaluation.

The standards are also needed to orient all new clinicians to the health agency. To facilitate the orientation of clinicians the standards should be imbedded into every policy, job description, and form used for documentation. Clinicians should receive a copy of the standards as well as the policies to review *before* beginning their work at the new agency, with the expectation that they will implement the standards for all patients. During orientation the new clinicians need to be informed about their role in implementing the standards and data collection concerning patient outcomes. If mentors are available in the agency, the mentors should assist new clinicians in implementing the standards.

A standards committee should be established for each health discipline as well as a multidisciplinary practice committee. The function of these committees is to review the standards on a timely basis and communicate any changes throughout the organization, such as policies, job descriptions, etc.

DOCUMENTATION

When the standards have been written for a procedure/unit of care, the requirements for documentation have been defined. Standards facilitate the documentation of clinicians because standards specify what must be recorded about the patients' care and their responses to it. The standards not only cue clinicians concerning what must be documented but also can prevent duplication.

The design of the documentation reflects the policies of the organization and the requirements of the legal counsel for the organization. In many agencies clinicians are required to duplicate documentation on multiple forms in the patient's record. The author has observed in some agencies that "a clinician has to record the same information seven times on multiple forms in the patient's record."[21] It appears that when a new form is added to the patient's record, the form it was designed to replace remains on the record. A result is that the patient's record grows and the time required to document patient care increases significantly. The clinicians' time is very valuable; therefore, *they should not be required to document anything more than once.*

In addition, the format of the standards has to meet the requirements of accrediting agencies and third-party payers such as Medicare and insurance companies. Third-party payers are now requiring the documentation by clinicians of all equipment and supplies used in care for which the agency can receive reimbursement. Because these requirements vary among companies and from state to state, administrators need to know the requirements for documentation that affect their organization. For example, in the past a complicated wound dressing might require 20 minutes to complete, including documentation. Now, because the number of gauze squares, cotton balls, and other reimbursable items used in the dressing must be documented, it requires 25 minutes to complete the procedure.

There is increasing complexity of patients' care and increased documentation required; concomitantly, there is no increase in the number of clinicians. There needs to be a way to decrease the time required for documentation. Otherwise, clinicians may have to choose between implementing care and documenting it.

Formatted text can contain the standards, including the requirements of outside agencies, and still permit the clinician to individualize the care for patients. This type of text can be easily updated and can decrease the time clinicians spend on documentation. Because the formatted text is easy to read clinicians may require less time for the exchange of information. Formatting can be used for consistency and decreased time required for:

a. Assessing patients
b. Designing plans of care
c. Documenting the standards implemented
d. Evaluation of patient outcomes

For example, with formatted text, it is possible to create a plan of care for a patient in less than 3 minutes that might have required 30 minutes of a clinician's time. It is possible to format parts of reports/consultations, reducing the amount of text required to be written by the clinician. The formatting can include the supplies and equipment required to implement a unit of care to reduce the time required to document these items. It is possible to obtain a formatted form that can be used to evaluate the patient's progress related to her specific needs in less than 3 minutes.

When clinicians have tools that they can use to facilitate the care they provide and still meet the requirements of accreditating agencies and third-party payers, they can focus their attention on identifying health problems/patient care needs, implementing the standards of care related to those problems/needs, and evaluating the patient's progress/responses to the interventions.

IMPLEMENTING STANDARDS IN AN INTERDISCIPLINARY TEAM

After the interdisciplinary units of care have been designed and tested for validity, they are ready to be implemented by the health team. The standards must be woven into the communication as well as the documentation by members of the health team. The quality of communication processes among health professionals significantly affects the quality of care the patient experiences because most patients need the skills of more than one health professional in assessing their health status, designing and implementing the plan of care, and evaluating the quality of patient outcomes. In many agencies the following pattern of information flow could ensure positive outcomes for patients in an organization embracing quality management.

INITIAL ASSESSMENT

On admission, one of the health team members, usually a nurse, assesses the patient and designs the patient's first plan of care. This plan is implemented until the first interdisciplinary team meeting unless the patient's needs/problems change; if there is a change, a modified plan is implemented.

It is recommended that *before the interdisciplinary conference every member of the health team do an assessment of the patient.* This assessment contains the content standards for assessment related to the identification of problems/needs that can be addressed by each health discipline (see chapter 4, section 1). (In some agencies all the health team members do not assess the patient to identify what patient care needs or problems should be addressed on the patient's plan of care. When this occurs, there is an inadequate assessment concerning the patient, resulting in a plan of care that does not meet *all* the patient's health problems or needs). A complete assessment also can decrease the time required to plan the patient's care in the planning conference because the health team has all the information required to plan the patient's care.

INTERDISCIPLINARY PLANNING

The interdisciplinary team meetings are "goal directed consisting of *all* health professionals involved with a specific patient's care."[22] A member of each health discipline presents the results of assessment. Because the standards of assessment have been implemented, there are no gaps or unnecessary duplication in the patient's data base.

After the patient's initial data base has been reviewed:

1. Interdisciplinary units of care related to the patient's needs and problems are placed on the patient's plan of care in order of their priority.

2. Units of care that are specific to a particular health discipline can be added to the plan.

3. Units of care can be individualized to meet the patient's specific needs and are coordinated with the resources available at the agency or at other agencies by referral.

4. Each discipline identifies the components of the plan for which it has responsibility; that is, the interventions and the patient outcomes that clinicians will assess to determine the patient's progress.

5. The coordinator of the plan must be identified to ensure that all components of the plan are being implemented as designed.
6. The plan is printed (with a computer system) or written (manual system).

In summary, when all members of the team have a descriptive mental picture of the needs of the patient, the plan of care they design is individualized to meet the specific needs/problems of the patient. Copies of the plan are kept by each discipline participating in the patient's care. These copies can be reviewed to ensure the interventions are being implemented and the outcomes are being evaluated in a timely fashion. If clinicians are using the plan to document the patient's progress, the formatting of the text is related to what must be documented for each unit of care.

IMPLEMENTATION OF THE PLAN

Each clinician implements the interventions for which he or she is responsible, collects data on the patient's progress toward the outcomes, and documents the patient's progress and the responses to all interventions on the patient record.

EVALUATION OF THE QUALITY OF PATIENT OUTCOMES

Evaluation of patient outcomes should be done *for every patient* using the outcome standards related to the patient's plan of care. For example, in acute care the time frame for the evaluation of care may be daily or every 2 to 3 days in less acutely ill patients. In long-term care, evaluation should be done at least weekly to identify the progress of the patient in relation to long-term goals. The evaluation of the patient's progress can occur during every visit to a patient in her home or during every appointment in a clinic or other community agency. (See evaluation method in section 2.)

ADDITIONAL INTERDISCIPLINARY CONFERENCES

When a clinician or coordinator identifies a significant change in the patient's health status, or when the outcomes related to the units of care on the patient's plan of care should be positive, another interdisciplinary conference is held. Before the conference each health team member should evaluate the patient's health status using the patient outcomes for which they are responsible as well as the items listed on the total assessment they do for each new patient. This is done to identify the patient's progress toward the outcomes and to identify new problems/needs the patient is experiencing. During the conference the patient's plan of care is updated, priorities are identified, and responsibilities for implementing the plan are assigned.

An innovative interdisciplinary approach to the implementation of valid and efficient interdisciplinary units of care is case management and managed care. **Case management and managed care** are "clinical systems that focus care on the attainment of appropriate patient outcomes within effective and efficient time lines and resource consumption."[23] "In managed care, the standards of care are established with concurrent and ongoing review using the standards."[24] Variance from the standard is identified and promptly addressed for the individual patient. The variance identified for a group of patients with the same unit of care is aggregated for retrospective review.

One of the components of case management is the use of critical paths.[25] Critical paths outline the expected time frame (valid outcome standards) and interventions/observations (valid and efficient process and content standards) that have been defined for the care of a population of patients. The time lines and resources are incorporated in the critical paths established by all the members of the health team. Then the outcomes of care are stated in measurable terms. Incorporated into the outcomes are the length of stay, cost, and patient satisfaction.[26]

The members of the health team use the critical paths to guide the implementation of the patient's plan of care and to identify situations in which the patient is deviating from the critical path (variance). Variance can be caused by the system, clinician, and patient. System-related variance is caused by a problem in the health agency, such as equipment breakdown, slow turnaround of tests, or not enough extended-care beds in the community to permit patients to be discharged. Variance related to clinicians occurs when members of the health team fail to order a test or procedure essential to the patient's discharge, or when patients do not reach expected outcomes. Patient-related variances are defined by characteristics within the patient, such as age or lack of family support.[27] Patient variance from the critical paths is addressed when clinicians exchange information within a health discipline, interdisciplinary planning meetings, or one-to-one communication between members of the health team.

The progress of the patient is evaluated at the time defined in the outcome standards.[28] In addition, aggregate variance, that is, the cumulative variance that occurs among patients within specified types or between case types must be analyzed to identify what patterns emerge.[29] Positive patient outcomes are measured in quality of care, length of stay, and resource utilization.

In case management, care is directed by a case manager who is a primary nurse with the responsibility for:

1. Developing outcomes for a caseload of patients
2. Working with the patient and health care team to accomplish those outcomes. The case manager has accountability for an appropriate length of stay, the effective use of resources, and meeting established standards.[30]

With methodologies like case management in place, the clinicians are able to "prospectively plan for care and, in turn, measure the effectiveness of this collaborative plan."[31]

Clinicians need assistance from administrators in removing barriers to improving the quality of care and the correct number and mix of staff to ensure positive outcomes for patients. Thus, standards need to be imbedded into the work of administrators.

EMBEDDING STANDARDS INTO THE WORK OF ADMINISTRATORS

One of the major assignments of managers in health care organizations is to implement staffing and costing methodologies. Because the results of these methodologies should be positive patient outcomes, staffing and costing strategies should be based on standards.

Staffing is the assignment of the correct number of staff with appropriate qualifications to implement the standards of care on each patient's plan of care. Staffing results from the identified costs of care when patient outcomes are positive.

Total labor costs include the time by level of clinician required to implement the standards of care for each patient (direct care) as well as other activities done by staff in the clinical setting (indirect care).

Valid and efficient standards determine the combinations of interventions and observations that result in positive outcomes for patients. When clinicians have enough time and are committed to implement standards of care, patients do not experience complications; acuity levels and length of stay are decreased, resulting in lower costs of care. And clinicians, knowing they are providing care that produces positive outcomes for patients, will experience satisfaction in their work.

Staffing and budgeting should result from the interaction between cost control and quality control. "Cost control is the financial expense allocated only for what is necessary and appropriate." "Quality control refers to the development of and compliance with established standards of practice."[32] Thus, administrators need to identify the factors that increase as well as decrease the costs of care. After the significant factors are identified, strategies can be implemented to control costs.

One of the most common approaches to staffing and the costs of care is the use of a Patient Classification System. Although there is variation among the Patient Classifiction Systems, the process of patient classification involves the prediction of care requirements using critical indicators within a group of [category] for a specified period of time.[33] The clinician is required to check off various activities and procedures (critical indicators) according to the frequency of their occurrence during the care of the patient during a specific period of time. A patient is placed into a category according to perceived time requirements.[34]

A different approach is the Individual Patient type of costing/staffing system.[35] This method uses the actual time required to implement interventions/ observations (valid and efficient standards) on each patient's plan of care multiplied by the cost of the clinician who implemented the standards to identify staffing and labor costs.[36]

VALIDITY OF THE METHOD

An important consideration when selecting a costing/staffing methodology is the method's validity and reliability.

Validity of the method for identifying staffing needs and labor costs should be established to provide administrators with accurate data required for decision making; the time/costs related to the implementation of care must accurately reflect the care implemented. Some methods are based on the assumption that a particular activity or task takes the same amount of time, on average, regardless of other patient characteristics or needs.[37] *Duration, intensity, and/or complexity of patient care requirements are not included.*[38]

Other methods are based on the premise that the costs should result from the *actual time required for the implementation of the standards designed to meet each patient's needs.*[39]

Timing studies related to care activities should include the time required to implement the standards of care.[40] If the timing studies do not measure the actual time required to implement standards of care, the quality dimension will be omitted in the cost; there will not be enough staff to implement the standards of care. Thus, the method used in the timing studies should be evaluated to ensure that the standards are being implemented *before* the timings are done.

Some methods for identifying the cost of staffing and care rely on establishing the *average amount of care by a patient category.* If the number of categories is small, a limitation will exist in variability of the data, which will not provide accurate data for identifying the costs of care.[41] To avoid the problems associated with categories, the staffing and the cost of care is derived for *each* patient.[42]

Skill mix is an important dimension to include in costing or staffing methodologies. If the relationship between the level of staff and hours of care is undefined, the relationship between level of staff and the cost of care is also undefined.[43] When the level of staff required to implement the standards for each cluster of interventions and observations is specified, the costs *accurately reflect the level of staff implementing the standards of care.*[44]

The frequency with which data related to the needs of patients is collected can also affect both staffing and costing. For example, the time required for implementing the standards can vary from shift to shift or from one home/clinic visit to another based on the changing needs of the patient. Thus, the method must be flexible enough to identify the current needs of the patients.[45]

RELIABILITY OF THE METHOD

The reliability of the tools and the consistency of the data collectors are crucial to the validity of the system that determines the cost of care. For example, it is assumed that nurses accurately and honestly complete forms containing lists of activities that determine the staffing as well as costing. When clinicians select activities being experienced by patients, there is a tendency to "ensure" there is enough staff by selecting those activities with the highest score.[46] In other methods the staffing and costing result from the time required to implement the standards on each patient's current plan of care.[47]

INDIRECT CARE

Indirect care activities are numerous unit/facility-specific activities, some patient-related and some unrelated to direct patient care, that clinicians do in addition to the care of the patients.[48] Indirect care activities can be categorized as those activities related to a specific patient's care, activities related to the work of other departments, and/or personal activities. [49] The indirect care values reflect "unit-specific activities that are defined, quantified, and assigned a skill level," which is added to each patient's direct care to determine the total cost for the patient.[50] Because the amount of time spent on indirect care varies from unit to unit, the indirect care time needs to be established for each clinical unit. For clinicians providing care to patients in their homes, travel time is an indirect care variable that affects the number of patients that can be visited each day.

REPORTS

In order to implement standards in a valid and reliable staffing/costing methodology that enables administrators to make rapid and effective decisions when changes need to be made, the following types of reports should be available:

1. Time/labor costs of care by staff class for a clinical unit or home visit by specific period of time (shift/week/home visit/clinic visit)
   a. Direct care
   b. Indirect Care
   c. Total care[51,52,53]

2. The time/costs of each patient's care, as well as length of stay, can be compared to the results of the evaluation of care for patients with the same patient care needs from clinical unit to clinical unit; from one multidisciplinary team to another; from one clinic to another; and, for patients receiving home care, from various community agencies. These reports assist in identifying the care that results in positive outcomes and that is also efficient.

3. A comparision of the units of care on the plans of care throughout a patient's stay with the patterns of other patients with the same patient care needs to determine the most effective and efficient patterns.

4. An identification of those complications that are preventable in the patients' plans of care and comparison of the costs of care of patients who experienced complications with those who experienced positive outcomes.

There are many characteristics of the methods used to identify costs and for staffing. The major difference is that "staffing is predictive; that is, data are obtained before the care is provided. The data related to labor costs must reflect *the care that has been implemented*." [54]

In some methodologies the data related to the staffing and costing are the same; thus, the costs of care are collected *before* the care is rendered. In summary, when implementing a method for staffing and identifying the labor costs of care, to ensure positive outcomes for patients, the method should be valid and reliable with standards as the method's major component.

In addition to the effect of standards on staffing and costing methodologies, standards should be reflected in the job descriptions and policies of all departments in the organization.

JOB DESCRIPTIONS AND POLICIES

Frequently, job descriptions and policies are confused with standards of care. One reason for this is that there are various definitions in the literature for each of these concepts. The first step in implementing job descriptions and policies, therefore, is to write a definition of them. One definition of a **job description** is a written statement listing the qualifications and the major responsibilities of an individual who holds a specific position in the organization. The major purpose of a job description is to provide a person unfamiliar with a job a brief but accurate picture of what a person holding the job does. Examples of statements in a job description include:

1. Implements the standards of care for patients assigned to her
2. Is responsible for planning the assignments of all other personnel on the clinical unit when assigned as charge nurse
3. Participates in the assessment, planning, implementation, and evaluation as a member of the health team
4. Is responsible for orientation of new staff to the unit/agency

A job description should include a description of the performance outcomes expected if an individual fulfills the responsibilities of her position. For those responsibilities related to the implementation of the standards of care, the outcome standards of the procedures/units of care for those patients receiving care from this clinician are the performance standards. For the additional responsibilities of clinicians, other performance criteria are used to evaluate their performance. For example:

Responsibility	*Performance Criteria*
Orientation of new staff to the unit	Content of the orientation includes physical layout of the unit, unit policies, emergency procedures, standards of care.

While job descriptions are helpful in orienting new staff to their responsibilities, they need to be written so that as changes are made in the reponsibilities of staff related to quality improvement, the changes can easily be made in the job descriptions.

A **policy** is a written statement that clearly describes the responsibility and actions to be taken in a given set of circumstances. A policy provides directions for decision making for a specific purpose so that action can be taken within the framework of the organization's mission and goals. Policies are written to protect the safety of patients and for the legal protection of the staff in an organization, but the scope of policies vary from one organization to another. For example, policies can define the hours to be worked, permitted absences, as well as rules for visitors. Policies also specify *who* can implement standards of care in a specific situation. The details of *what* is to be done in a patient situation are defined by process and content standards. For example, policies, as well as standards, are developed for the following interventions/units of care and who can implement them.

- *Administration of Intravenous Chemotherapy*
- *Vaginal Delivery*
- *Informed Consent*

For the intervention *Defibrillation*, note the difference between a policy and a process standard:

Policy	*Process Standard*
Only clinicians who have completed the prescribed instruction and passed the competency exam can defibrillate a patient.	All personnel should stand clear of the patient and the patient's bed during defibrillation.
(Defines the qualifications of staff that can do this procedure.)	(Defines what must be done during this procedure.)

Thus, a policy provides directions for decision making in a given situation, while process and content standards define what interventions and observations should be implemented.

In organizations implementing quality management it is important that standards be woven into all aspects of administrative decision making to ensure that patients experience positive outcomes.

Now proceed to section 2, "Evaluation of the Quality of Care."

SECTION 2

Evaluation of the Quality of Care

A vital department in the organization whose mission is quality improvement is the one responsible for the evaluation of patient outcomes. The responsibilities of this department are the evaluation of the quality of patient outcomes and recommendations for change in the organization. "The ultimate reason for measuring quality is to maintain and improve the quality of care."[55,56] The results of the evaluation of care should have the highest priority for administrative decision making because changes must be initiated, when indicated, to improve clinical practice.[57]

Although every clinician and administrator can agree with the need for the evaluation of care, the following issues must be addressed before beginning the evaluation program:

1. Validity of the data
2. Reliability of the method
3. Type and source of data
4. Scope of the data collection

VALIDITY

A major function of a quality improvement program is to provide valid and reliable data regarding outcomes of patient care.[58] The outcomes should be designed to indicate the patient's progress, or lack of it, toward the goals of care (see chapter 3). Each cluster of patient outcomes is a "photograph" of the patient at a point in time after experiencing care related to a specific problem/diagnosis/need. (see chapter 3). The text of the outcomes provides the clarity and detail of the photograph.

Patient outcomes should contain the following characteristics (see chapter 3):

1. A specific description of the impact of care on the patient
2. An outcome specifically related to standards defining the care
3. A description understood by the persons evaluating care
4. A time when the outcome can be observed
5. The nurse's responsibility in relation to the outcome
6. Validity of the outcomes

The outcome standards for both procedures and units of care are used to determine the quality of care that patients receive. The validity of the standards must be established before beginning to evaluate the quality of the care; there must be a direct relationship between the outcomes of care and the data that are collected during the evaluation process (see chapter 7).

After the validity of the standards has been established, there are two additional questions that must be answered before beginning to evaluate care:

- How many patients must be sampled to determine whether a specified quality of care is being rendered?
- What percent of patients must have positive outcomes for the care to be at a specified quality?

In some methods of evaluation, the results obtained using a statistical sample assume the sample of patients is representative of the entire population of patients receiving care related to a specified set of standards.[59]

In quality management, every patient's care is evaluated while the patient is receiving care. This evaluation is done at the critical points in time when a clinician could intervene to reverse a pattern of outcomes that might result in complications or an extended stay in the institution.

In some methods a benchmark percent of those patients, regardless of the size of the sample, experiencing positive outcomes equals a desirable level of quality. For example, if the benchmark is set at 85%, and 85 % of the patients in the sample have positive outcomes, health professionals believe that quality care has been provided for the entire population of the patients in that facility.

In quality management it is expected that all the patients experience positive outcomes. Because the methodology for collecting data is woven into the clinician's work, it is possible to collect outcome data on all patients to monitor their progress while the patients are receiving care. Thus, if a patient is not progressing, the clinicians can change the patient's plan of care and implement interventions while the patient is receiving care to ensure positive outcomes.

RELIABILITY

To ensure reliability of the data collection, those persons gathering the data must be able to consistently implement the method as well as be able to accurately recognize the patient outcomes.[60] Observations can be faulty when observers are poorly trained, misinterpret what is occurring, or observe activities at the wrong time.

Clinicians must participate in the development and ownership of the standards, as well as collecting and evaluating patient data.[61] When the outcomes for a specific patient are woven into the implementation of standards of care, clinicians can collect outcome data as part of their care of the patient.

SOURCES OF DATA

A temptation of evaluators is to collect everything and anything related to quality.[62] Volumes of data are often saved for "accreditation purposes," but few of these data will ensure quality care for patients presently receiving care.

One approach is to list all the Quality Management activities in an agency, such as minutes of meetings, circulation of files in the library, organizational charts, and administrative reports. While these data are needed to demonstrate there is an operational Quality Management program, they do not directly demonstrate that quality care is being provided for patients.[63]

One source of data commonly used to measure the success of a Quality Management program is the number of studies completed as compared to the number completed in a previous time period.[64] Merely counting the number of monitors, however, provides no information on the appropriateness of the studies, nor does it provide information regarding the quality of care.[65]

A common method used to evaluate patient outcomes is to read clinician's documentation of the outcomes in the patient's record. While it is important to review clinicians' documentation at periodic intervals to identify whether their charting is accurate and pertinent, the documentation should not be the primary source of evaluation of patient outcomes. Many patients experience postive outcomes that are not documented. If clinicians have not consistently documented the outcomes they have observed, reviewing charts can be very frustrating and time consuming because data is missing. Evaluation of the quality of care may be impossible. In addition, because there is a time lag between when patient outcomes are documented and the review of the documentation, the opportunity may be lost for a clinician to intervene early enough to ensure positive outcomes for a patient.

The source of data for evaluation of the care should be the patient or clinical data that define the outcomes of care.[66] (See chapter 3.)

PATIENT SATISFACTION

No evaluation of care would be complete without the evaluation of patient/family satisfaction. As Bader states, "Patients often judge the institution's quality by the quality of clinical services."[67] Patients cannot evaluate the quality of all dimensions of nursing care, but they can provide valuable feedback to clinicians about their approach to patients and families (see chapter 3). Patient satisfaction is a subjective view that caregivers must regard as reality.[68] The patient's perspective completes the picture of the quality of care.[69] Also, the clinician's approach to the patient/family can positively or negatively affect the patient's outcomes. Therefore, patient/family satisfaction should be included in the evaluation of patient outcomes.

The time frame for obtaining patient/family satisfaction data is an important consideration. If patient satisfaction data related to their care while admitted is obtained after discharge, it will be difficult, if not impossible, to change a patient's negative view of clinicians and the institution. Data related to patient/family satisfaction should be obtained as the patients proceed through the phases of their care. Because open communication between clinicians and the patient/family usually results in a positive relationship, the patient's/family's opinion can change even if at first it was negative. As Petersen states, "Dissatisfied patients can be won back into our favor."[70]

Because of the importance of the consumer's evaluation of care, patient/family satisfaction should be evaluated while the patient is experiencing care to identify whether the needs of the patient and family are being met (see chapter 3). For example, the patient's family may stay for long periods during the day with a patient who is terminally ill. They are scared because their loved one is dying and are very hesitant to ask for anything that might increase their own comfort during the long hours they wait. If a clinician or patient/family advocate inquires about their needs, family members might express them. When family members are comfortable, they can provide more support for the patient. And as an additonal benefit to the facility, they will tell others about the kindness of the clinicians to the patient and themselves.

It is also essential that some patients are contacted after discharge, such as when they have had to make adjustments in their lifestyle because of a health problem or are recovering from surgery or regarding the results of patient teaching. Using telephone call-backs, clinicians can receive direct information from the discharged patient about her current physical status and problems. The patient also can receive additional information related to her questions. Call-backs can facilitate problem solving after an early discharge and decrease liability for staff and health care facility.[71]

Now that some of the major factors affecting evaluation of care have been discussed, the methodology of evaluation will be presented.

METHODOLOGY

The evaluation method needs to be efficient as well as effective because of the diminishing resources available to health care organizations. In addition, the method should have a scope to identify all types of health problems and include outcomes that point to the corrective action that should be employed when early negative outcomes occur.

The evaluation method should contain the following types of data collection:

1. Observation of the patient
2. Evaluation of the care of individual patients
3. Evaluation of the care of groups of patients with similiar diagnoses

When these types of data collection are implemented, the results not only indicate whether positive outcomes are being experienced by patients but that the results also point to the corrective action that might be needed if negative outcomes are beginning to occur.

OBSERVATION OF THE PATIENT

The first type of data collection is the systematic observation done by clinicians when providing care. Because clinicians need to focus on the patient outcomes to identify the patient's responses to care, the expected outcomes are listed on each patient's plan of care as observations. Thus, as the care is provided, the clinician is also monitoring patient outcomes.

The outcome standards for both procedures and units of care are used to determine the quality of care that patients receive. Clinicians observe for the outcomes related to a specific procedure or unit of care. They compare the patient's responses to the outcome standards to ensure that they have implemented the care precisely and that the patient is experiencing positive outcomes. The observations help the clinicians make changes in the care as they are implementing the procedure based on the patient's responses. When patient outcomes can be included in the patient's plan of care and observed by clinicians as they do the care, an initial, vital component of the evaluation process is being implemented.

EVALUATION OF THE CARE OF INDIVIDUAL PATIENTS

Data are collected using the outcome standards for all the units of care that are on the patient's plan of care at the specific point in time when the outcomes should be achieved (defined by the outcome standards). For example, when a surgical patient is receiving care to prevent a complication such as pneumonia, clinicians should be making the observations daily to identify if the patient is experiencing any symptoms that could predispose to pneumonia. If a patient begins to experience any symptoms that could result in this complication, therapy can begin immediately to prevent this complication.

The time for the evaluation of the impact of the entire plan of care on the patient is done when the expected outcomes should be present. For example, as the patient progresses postoperatively, the outcome standards are used to evaluate the patient's progress (or lack of it). If the patient has not reached the positive outcomes usually reached by other patients at this day in their postoperative course, the clinicians must make a decision after they have answered the following questions:

- If the present plan of care is continued for another day, will the patient reach the expected outcomes for today?

- Can the plan of care be modified to improve the patient's progress toward the expected outcomes?

If the clinicians believe that in one more day the patient will progress satisfactorily, observations need to be made frequently during this 24-hour period to identify whether the patient is progressing or whether action should be taken to assist the patient. For example, the clinicians are teaching the patient about her care at home. The patient is not making satisfactory progress in learning the new changes in her lifestyle. The patient is experiencing mild anxiety. As the clinicians observe the patient during the next 24 hours, the patient's anxiety increases steadily so that she can no longer focus on what she needs to learn. When this is recognized by the accurate observation of a clinician, the unit of care *Moderate Anxiety* is added to the patient's plan of care and interventions are implemented to:

a. Identify the cause
b. Decrease the patient's anxiety until again she can focus on what she needs to learn

Now let's look at other examples of the evaluation of the impact of the plan of care on the patient. *For patients with chronic illness who have long-term goals*, the outcome standards related to their plan of care are used to evaluate the patient's status at *sequential points in time* to ensure:

1. The patient is progressing satisfactorily
2. The patient is not experiencing complications
3. The goals related to the needs of the patient's family are being met

Currently, it is required that the care of patients in most long-term care facilities be evaluated every 30 to 90 days. For many patients, this time period is not frequent enough to ensure that the goals of care are being met.

If a patient is terminally ill, evaluation of the patient's health status is done to prevent complications, ensure comfort, and provide the support and resources needed by both the patient and family. The specific time for evaluation is defined by when the expected, positive outcomes of each of the units of care on the patient's plan of care should occur.

For patients coming to an outpatient clinic, the outcome standards related to the patient's plan of care can be used to evaluate the patient's progress and/or the knowledge/skills the patient needs to cope with her illness *at every visit*. This is essential to identify factors in the patient's home situation that might be impeding the patient's coping with her health problem(s).

A component of each *home visit* should be an evaluation of the patient's status using the outcome standards on her plan of care. Many changes can occur to the patient between visits. Thus, an evaluation of the patient's progress at each visit is essential to ensure the patient experiences positive outcomes.

If negative outcomes begin to occur in any of these situations, the process standards associated with these outcomes can be used to assist in the identification of what needs to be changed to prevent this complication or lack of progress from occurring.

EVALUATION OF THE CARE OF GROUPS OF PATIENTS

When negative outcomes related to *one* unit of care are occurring for *more than one* patient, the outcome standards for that unit of care should be used to evaluate the outcomes of every patient experiencing this unit of care in the facility. This is done to identify if something has changed in the process of implementing care since the validity of the standards was established that changed the results from positive to negative outcomes.

For example, a unit of care was written for the procedure *Continuous Tube Feedings*. One of the outcome standards for this procedure was *the patient is not experiencing diarrhea*. When a patient experienced diarrhea on one of the clinical units, the outcome standards for this procedure were used to look at the health status of all patients who were receiving *Continuous Tube Feedings*. The results showed that 60% of the patients were experiencing diarrhea. Upon review of the process standards and the way the standards were being implemented, it was determined that the size of the bags holding the nutrients used in the tube feedings was changed from a small to large bag. The bag was hanging much longer than usual before being changed. Thus, the contents of the bag had begun to deteriorate, causing diarrhea in the patients. When the smaller bags were again used, no patients experienced diarrhea.

In another example, the rate of wound infection increased on a surgical oncology unit over a few months to a level much higher than any other clinical unit in the facility. Over 50% of the patients on this unit experienced a wound infection within their first three postoperative days. The process standards for *Wound Care* were used to evaluate the technique of every health professional that implemented that procedure. The results indicated that a new group of students who had not learned how to use sterile technique when changing a dressing were doing such things as:

1. Not using gloves or washing their hands between patients
2. Using the same set of gloves to change the dressings of all the patients

Obviously, these students did not implement the process standards for *Wound Care.* The cause of the negative outcomes was easily identified because, if valid process standards are implemented, positive outcomes result for patients.

DATA ANALYSIS

If the data are collected on forms similar to figure 7.1 in chapter 7, the data can be analyzed as explained in chapter 7.

SUMMARY

It is essential that the evaluation method you use to determine whether patients are receiving quality care should be valid and reliable, focus on patient outcomes by collecting data from the patient, and large enough in scope to quickly identify trends in negative outcomes. The data analysis method should be practical, providing results rapidly in easily understood reports that will facilitate recommendations for change when change is required.

SECTION 3
Quality Improvement

Every organization needs a quality improvement team with the authority as well as the responsibility to implement change when it is needed to improve the quality of the patient's outcomes. Because every person in the organization is a potential contributor to problems interfering with the quality of the organization, there should be representatives from every group in the organization on the quality improvement team.[72]

All team members must understand the values related to quality improvement and express the enthusiasm and endurance to proceed even when resistance occurs.[73] The team should comprise individuals who can clear roadblocks for those making changes.[74]

The purpose of the team is to identify and eliminate problems forever.[75] It is to "guide the improvement process and help it along."[76] Thus, the focus is not to just fix what went wrong in one situation but to eliminate the barriers creating the problem for the future. The approach to problem resolution is one of facing problems openly without searching for individuals to blame.[77]

Some examples of problems that might need elimination in a health care organization include:

- Insufficient numbers of qualified staff to ensure positive outcomes for patients
- A lack of cooperation among administrators at any level in the organization or a change in patients' environment that disrupts the care patients receive
- Insufficient or unproductive communication among members of the health team; the sequencing of the interventions is not organized and the patient/family receive conflicting information from various members of the team
- Discharge planning is not implemented by the entire team. A referral is not sent or the text of the referral is incomplete; the result is that a patient does not receive any visits from a community agency for a week after discharge.
- Placement of patients not available in the community
- Types of referrals accepted by community agencies unknown
- Criteria for acceptance at health care agencies unknown
- Third-party payer coverage for therapy/care needed but not provided
- Departments such as x-ray or EEG overbooked or closed
- Equipment breakdown
- Lab results' turnaround time is too long[78]

The organization that implements quality management or quality improvement will have the following characteristics:

1. Effective, efficient standards of care throughout the organization
2. Methods for making rapid change in the organization when needed
3. Productive communication processes throughout the organization
4. Reward systems for rewarding personnel when they make changes that facilitate the improvement of the quality of care as well as when patients are consistently experiencing positive outcomes
5. Valid and efficient methods for evaluating the quality of patient outcomes
6. Incentives for everyone in the organization to espouse quality and contribute to it

7. A compulsion to "beg for, demand innovation from everybody"[79]

8. Frequent change will require in all staff an "increased capacity to accept disruption"[80]

9. Removal of barriers to the pride of workmanship[81]

10. Emphasis on working together rather than focusing on individual performance

11. Emphasis on striving for improvement rather than setting thresholds of improvement

12. Emphasis is on self-evaluation and process improvement rather than inspection[82]

13. Effective communication by management to make it easier for employees to do their jobs

14. Celebration of the "small wins that are indicative of the solid day-to-day performance turned in by 90 percent of your work force"[83]

15. Coordination and integration of processes; coordination and integration requires the attention of the managerial and clinical leaders of the hospital[84]

16. Employee involvement in strategic planning sessions[85]

17. Implementation of computerized systems to rapidly compile comparative data related to quality/costs and to facilitate documentation for clinicians

18. Emphasis on a quality improvement team with the authority, as well as the responsibility, for innovating change[86]

19. Involvement of all persons at all levels in all functions of quality improvement[87]

The organization embracing quality management will need to be innovative in its approach to solving problems affecting the quality of patient outcomes. Most innovation will demand that historically adversarial relations

- Between various functions in the organization
- Between labor and management
- Between community agencies and the organization
- Between staff and consumer

be changed to cooperative.[88]

Conflict situations will need to be identified as opportunities for creative change.[89] Administrators in many organizations will need to change their style of leadership. As Dixon states, "The Continuous Quality Improvement approach develops leadership and teamwork from the point of service up, not administration down. Shared leadership requires administrators to take risks on other people's decisions, powers of persuasion, and competencies."[90] To comfort those administrators who may be nervous about beginning quality improvement in their organization, Peters states, "There are no limits to the ability to contribute on the part of a properly selected, well-trained, appropriately supported, and above all, committed person."[91]

There are some positive results for those who participate in quality improvement. Crosby explains: "Everything improves when an organization becomes genuinely involved in the quality improvement process. The lowering of the hassle level is one of the most pleasant side effects of the effort. Discussions are more orderly, and the problems of quality are resolved without emotion. Administrative actions become smoother, paperwork is less cumbersome. Longstanding confusion over procedures and processes is ironed out."[92]

In summary, the commitment of everyone working in a health organization must concern quality management. Crosby states that "the performance standard must be 'zero defects,' not 'that's close enough.'"[93] The cornerstone of quality management or quality improvement is the standards of care. The following saying by an anonymous author sums up this author's thoughts on quality management:

Every job is a self-portrait of the person who did it. Autograph your work with excellence! —*Anonymous*

NOTES

1. Joint Commission on Accreditation of Health Care Organizations. *Accreditation manual for hospitals*, p.138. Illinois: JCAHO, 1992.

2. Kritchevsky, S.B., and Simmons, B.P. "Continuous quality improvement: Concepts and applications for physical care," *Journal of the American Medical Association, 266*, p.1817, 1991.

3. Quality Watch. "Adopting Deming's quality improvement ideas: A case study," *Hospitals*, p.58, July 1990.

4. Martin, C.A. NAQAP position paper: "The role of QI in health care QA," *Journal of Quality Assurance*, p.14, November/December 1990.

5. Katz, J., and Green, E. "The blueprint for quality management: The agenda for the future," *The Encyclopedia of Nursing Care Quality, II*, p.45.

6. Crosby, P.B. *Quality is free*, p.19. New York: New American Library, 1979.

7. Ibid., p.14.

8. Crosby, P.B. *Quality without tears*, p.64. New York: McGraw-Hill, 1984.

9. Peters, T. *Thriving on chaos*, pp.79–80. New York: Alfred A. Knopf, 1987.

10. Ibid., p.80.

11. O'Leary, D. "President's Column," *Joint Commission Perspectives*, 8 (½), pp.2–3.

12. Masters, F., and Schmele, J.A. "Total quality management: An idea whose time has come," *Journal of Nursing Quality Assurance*, 5 (4), p.15, 1991.

13. Deming, W.E. *Out of the crisis*, p.24. Cambridge, Mass.: Massachusetts Institute of Technology Center for Advanced Engineering Study, 1986.

14. Crosby, op.cit., 1979, p.19.

15. Peters, op.cit., p.80.

16. Ibid., p.71.

17. Crosby, op.cit., p.65, 1979.

18. Coyne, C., and Killian, M. "A system for unit-based monitors of quality of nursing care," *Journal of Nursing Administration*, 17 (1), p.26, 1987.

19. Katz and Green, op.cit., p.50.

20. Crosby, op.cit., p.65, 1979.

21. Mason, E.J. "Integrating standards into the decision making of nurse clinicians and nurse administrators: the excelcare system." In P. Schroeder (Ed.), *The encyclopedia of nursing care quality*, 2, p.79. Gaithersburg, Md.: Aspen Publishers, 1991.

22. "The center for case management," *Definition*, p.1. Boston, Mass., Spring 1989.

23. Bower, Kathleen. "Standards as a benchmark of the case management approach to care delivery." In Schroeder, Patricia, *The Encyclopedia of nursing care quality: Approaches to nursing standards*, 12, p.59. Aspen, Colo., 1991.

24. Ibid., p.59.

25. Ibid., p.60.

26. Ibid., p.60.

27. Ibid., p.61.

28. Ibid., p.67.

29. Ibid., p.68.

30. Etheridge, M.L., Zander, K., and Bower, K. *Nursing case management: Blueprint for transformation*. Boston, Mass.: The Center for Case Management, New England Medical Center Hospitals, p.1, 1988.

31. Wood, Rosemary, Gruber, Bailey, Olsen, Nancy, and Tilkemeier, Diane. "Managed care: The missing link in quality improvement," *Journal of Nursing Care Quality, 6* (4) p.60, 1992.

32. Yaws, J.Y., and Deruvo, S.S. "Utilization management: Improving patient care while maintaining cost control," *Journal of Nursing Quality Assurance, 3* (2), p.53, 1989.

33. De Groot, H.A. "Patient classification system evaluation: Part 2," *Journal of Nursing Administration, 19* (7), p.30, 1989.

34. Edwardson, S.R., and Giovannetti, P.B. "A review of cost-accounting methods for nursing services," *Nursing Economics, 5* (3), p.113, 1987.

35. Mason, E.J., and Daugherty, J.K. *Excelcare System Manual*, Verona, Penn.: Authors, 1993, p.16.

36. Mason and Daugherty, op.cit., p.31.

37. De Groot, H.A. "Patient classification system evaluation: Part 1," *Journal of Nursing Administration, 19* (6), p.31, 1989.

38. Mason, op.cit., p.91.

39. Mason and Daugherty, op.cit., p. 32.

40. Porter-O'Grady,T. "Strategic planning: Nursing practice in PPS," *Nursing Management, 16* (10), p.56, 1985.

41. Dijkers, M., and Paradise, T. "PCS: One system for both staffing and costing," *Nursing Management, 17* (1), p.27, 1986.

42. Mason and Daugherty, op.cit., p. 33.

43. Dijkers, op.cit., p.28.

44. Mason and Daugherty, op.cit., p.33.

45. Prescott, P. "DRG prospective reimbursement: The nursing intensity factor," *Nursing Management, 17* (1), p.46, 1986.

46. Farnham, Jo Ann, Maez-Rauzi, Vicky, and Conway, Karin. "Balancing assignments: A PCS for a step down unit," *Nursing Management, 23* (3), March 1993.

47. Mason and Daugherty, op.cit., p.93.

48. Mason, op.cit., p.93.

49. Mason and Daugherty, op.cit., p.38.

50. O'Connor, N. "Integrating patient classification with cost accounting," *Nursing Management, 19* (10), pp.27–29, 1988.

51. Silva and Aderholdt, op.cit., p.49.

52. Mason, op.cit., p.96.

53. New, N. "Quality measurement: Quick, easy and unit-based," *Nursing Management, 20* (10), p.50, 1989.

54. Smeltzer, C. "Evaluating a successful quality assurance program: The process," *Journal of Nursing Quality Assurance, 2* (4), p.1, 1988.

55. Ibid., p.7.

56. Ibid., p.4.

57. Ibid., p.7.

58. Wilson, C.K. "Developing a quality assurance program evaluation: A process model," *Journal of Nursing Quality Assurance, 2* (4), p.37, 1988.

59. Smeltzer, op.cit., p.7.

60. Wilson, op.cit., p.37.

61. Smeltzer, op.cit., p.3.

62. Wilson, op.cit., p.41.

63. Smeltzer, op.cit., p.3.

64. Wilson, op.cit., p.41.

65. Saum, M. "Evaluation: A vital component of the quality assurance program," *Journal of Nursing Quality Assurance, 2* (4), p.18, 1988.

66. Driever, M., and Birenbaum, L. "Patton's utilization-focused evaluation as a basis of the quality assurance process," *Journal of Nursing Quality Assurance, 2* (4), p.48.

67. Bader, M.M. "Nursing care behaviors that predict patient satisfaction," *Journal of Nursing Quality Assurance, 2* (3), p.12, 1988.

68. Megivern, Karen, Halm, Margo, and Jones, Gerry. "Measuring patient satisfaction as an outcome of nursing care," *Journal of Nursing Care Quality, 6* (4), July 1992.

69. Petersen, M.B.H. "Measuring patient satisfaction: Collecting useful data," *Journal of Nursing Quality Assurance, 2* (3), p.25, 1988.

70. Ibid.

71. Riley, J. "Telephone call-backs: Final patient care evaluation," *Nursing Management, 20* (9), pp.64–66, 1989.

72. Crosby, op.cit., p.152, 1979.
73. Crosby, op.cit., p.112, 1984.
74. Ibid., p.106.
75. Ibid., p.112.
76. Crosby, op.cit., p.106, 1979.
77. Crosby, op.cit. p.112, 1984.
78. Bower, op.cit., p.61, 1991.
79. Peters, op.cit., p.275.
80. Ibid., p.277.
81. Lopresti, John, and Whetstone, William, "Total quality manage-ment: Doing things right," *Nursing Management, 24* (1), p.35, January 1993.
82. Peters, op.cit., p.284.
83. Ibid., p.305.
84. Patterson, Carole H. "Joint commission nursing care standards: The framework for a comprehensive program to assess and improve qual-ity," *Journal of Nursing Care Quality, 7* (2), p.5, January 1993.
85. Peters, op.cit., p.284.
86. Ibid.
87. Ibid.
88. Ibid., p.278.
89. Fleeger, Mary Ann. "Assessing organizational culture: A planning strategy," *Nursing Management 24* (2), p.41, February 1993.
90. Dixon, Ingrid I. "Continuous quality improvement in shared leader-ship," *Nursing Management, 24* (1), p.40, January 1993.
91. Peters, op.cit., p.284.
92. Crosby, op.cit., p.84, 1984.
93. Ibid.

Appendix

INTRODUCTION

The appendix was added to this version of the book in order to provide additional examples of standards of care. The examples that have been included illustrate the use of standards in situations in which clinicians frequently ask for assistance in writing standards. The examples have been selected to illustrate an approach to writing units of care related to these clinical situations and/or how the units of care can be implemented in planning, implementing, and evaluating care. In addition, the format of the standards includes the requirements of some of the accrediting and reimbursement agencies. Lastly, the standards that will complete the examples of units of care throughout the book have been included in the appendix.

The sections of the appendix are examples of:

1. Writing Standards for the Care of Children
2. Writing Standards for Perioperative Care
3. Writing Standards for the Emergency Department
4. Writing Standards for Discharge Planning
5. Writing Standards for Home Care
6. Standards to Complete Examples in the Book

Now select any appendix and read the suggestions for writing and implementing standards with the accompanying examples.

SECTION 1
Writing Standards for the Care of Children

Inherent in the standards for the care of children are the standards related to each stage of growth and development. These standards define the essential interventions to be implemented for a child at a specific stage of growth and development. There are at least two approaches for writing the standards related to growth and development.

The first is including the standards for growth and development with other standards in a unit of care; for example, *Potential/Actual Suicide— Adolescent*. Some units of care are applicable to children in more than one stage of growth and development; for example, *Reactive Airway Disease*. In order to meet each child's growth and development needs, a unit of care is written for *each stage* of growth and development. When the child's plan of care is designed, the unit of care related to growth and development is added to the units of care identified during assessment.

The following examples will illustrate both ways of writing units of care containing the standards related to growth and development. The examples are:

1. Stresses of Hospitalization—Toddler[1]
2. Infant Admission Assessment[2]
3. Pain, Older Toddler/Preschooler[3]
4. Potential Suicide—Adolescent[4]

Also included in this section are some examples of units of care related to the health problems children experience but without the standards related to growth and development for each of the stages. When these units of care are added to the child's plan of care, a unit of care related to the child's growth and development stage must be added to the plan.

5. Reactive Airway Disease—Acute Stabilization Phase[5]
6. Reactive Airway Disease—Convalescent Phase[6]
7. Reactive Airway Disease—Parent Teaching[7]

As the title indicates, this unit of care contains the interventions related to the meeting the needs of a hospitalized toddler.

STRESSES OF HOSPITALIZATION—TODDLER

Goals

1. The toddler will experience minimal stress of hospitalization.
2. The toddler will experience minimal stress from separation from parents.
3. The parents will recognize the child's stress and attempt to comfort him.

Process Standards

1. Explain all procedures to parents/patient in terms they can understand.
2. Encourage one parent to stay overnight or visit as frequently as possible. Offer phone numbers to unit and encourage calls or call parents to update on child's status.
3. Encourage parents to keep security objects with the child (blanket, pacifier, favorite toys, family photos).
4. Try to maintain home regimes while infant is in the hospital (feeding times, nap time, play).
5. Support the parents when they must leave the child, as the child will usually scream and protest. Comfort the child by staying with him or her and engaging in diversional activities until he or she settles.
6. Identify and respond to toddler distress signals and offer soothing techniques, pain medication, etc.
7. Incorporate play into care-giving activities.
8. Tell parents to refrain from extra expectations of child during and immediately following hospitalization (toilet training).
9. Prepare the toddler for a painful procedure just prior to its being performed. Avoid the terms "shots" and other words that have negative meaning since procedure is necessary for child's health.
10. Allow toddler to play with safe equipment used in his or her treatment.
11. Allow toddler to express hurt/anger and encourage parents to comfort the child.
12. Refrain from talking about the child within earshot.
13. Support parents who notice regression in their child's behavior while hospitalized and explain that this is a normal toddler's reaction to stress.

Outcome Standards

At all times:

1. The toddler experiences minimal stress of hospitalization.*
2. The toddler experiences minimal stress from separation from parents.*
3. The parents recognize the child's stress and attempt to comfort him.

*As indicated by the child's behavior.

The next unit of care was designed as the admission assessment of the infant. As a result of implementing this unit of care, the infant's plan of care can be designed.

INFANT ADMISSION

Goals

1. The infant admission assessment will be accurate and complete.
2. The parents will be oriented to the clinical unit.

Process Standards

3. Prepare room.
   a. Appropriate crib, nonelectric bed, or electric bed
   b. Seating for parent or significant other
   c. Stand with appropriate personal hygiene items

4. Ensure that the ID band on the patient matches the admission paperwork.
5. Place weight in KG on bracelet.
6. Place allergy/sensitivity label on chart and Kardex as appropriate.
7. Orient patient/parents to:
   a. Review parent pamphlet
   b. Review visiting hours
   c. Obtain sleeper chair for parent who will be spending the night.
   d. Use of the call light
   e. Use of the crib or bed
   f. Reason for hospitalization and expectations in the next several hours

g. Policy for use of home electrical equipment

h. Location of playroom, lounge, coffee, etc.

6. Complete following assessment of patient and document information on database.

GENERAL INFORMATION

DOB:_____ Name:_____Nickname:_____Primary Language:_____
Person giving information:_____
Whom to notify in emergency:_____
Relationship:_____Home Phone:
                                     Work Phone:_____
Mode of Admission: ( ) Ambulatory ( ) Wheelchair ( ) Stretcher
                   ( ) Other:_____
Adm. Vitals: Temp:____ P:____ R:____ B/P:____ Ht:____Wt:____KG
Bloods:_____CXR:____ U/A:____ Other:_____
Parents understanding of Adm.:_____
Personal Meds.: ( ) None ( ) Sent to Pharmacy ( ) Sent Home
               ( ) At bedside with physician order:_____

GENERAL HISTORY

Allergies: Drugs:_____
           Food:_____Other:_____
Previous Hospitalizations:
Age:_____ Illness:_____Duration:_____
Medications taken at home:
Drug:_____Start Date:_____Last Dose:_____
Nutrition: ( ) Regular diet ( ) Diet_____
Appetite: ( ) Good ( ) Fair ( ) Poor
Food Group likes_____
Food Group dislikes:_____
History of present illness:_____

SOCIAL HISTORY

Family: ( ) Cardiac ( ) Hypertension ( ) Seizures ( ) Respiratory
( ) Diabetes ( ) Cancer ( ) Ulcers ( ) Other:_____

Primary Caregiver of Patient: ( ) Parents ( ) Single Parent
( ) Foster Parent ( ) Other:_____
Are both the parents at home? ( ) Yes ( ) No
If adopted, is child aware? ( ) Yes ( ) No
Visitation: ( ) Parent staying ( ) Parents can visit ( ) Other:_____
Sibling/pets at home: Name:_____Sex:_____Age:_____
Special social information (cultural, occupational, home situation)

IMMUNIZATIONS

	Up-to-date	Behind in vaccine	Disease: Yes	No
Hepatitis B	( )	_____	( )	( )
DPT	( )	_____	( )	( )
Polio	( )	_____	( )	( )
HIB	( )	_____	( )	( )
Chicken Pox	( )	_____	( )	( )

TB Test: ( ) Yes ( ) No When:_____( ) Not known
Exposure to communicable diseases over the past four weeks: ( ) No
( ) Yes:_____

ACTIVITIES OF DAILY LIVING

Bedtime____AM/PM ( ) No nap   Nap____AM/PM, Nap____AM/PM
Child sleeps in a : ( ) Bed ( ) Crib
Foods: ( ) Breast milk ( ) Formula: Type:_____
    ( ) Cereal_____( ) Fruit_____
    ( ) Vegs_____( ) Meats_____
    ( ) Strained food ( ) Junior food ( ) Finger food
    Drinks from a ( ) Cup ( ) Bottle   Pacifier: ( )Yes ( )No

PRESENT PHYSICAL FINDINGS

Respiratory:
( ) Retractions ( ) Nasal flaring ( ) Wheezing ( ) Stridor ( ) Grunt ( ) Periodic breathing/apnea ( ) Cyanosis ( ) Pallor ( ) Clear ( ) Congested ( ) I/E Wheeze ( ) Rales ( ) Rhonchi ( ) Cough

Cardiovascular:
( ) Tachycardia ( ) Bradycardia ( ) Chest pain ( ) Edema ( ) Bounding pulse
( ) History of murmur ( ) Murmur present ( ) Irregular rhythm

Mouth/Teeth/Gums:
( ) Braces ( ) Loose teeth ( ) Missing teeth ( ) Caries ( ) Odor ( ) Bleeding

Vision:
( ) No difficulty ( ) Blurred ( ) Diplopia ( ) Blind ( ) Glasses ( ) Contact lens
( ) Artificial eye

Hearing:
( ) No difficulty ( ) Limited ( ) Deaf ( ) Tinnitus ( ) Hearing aid

Speech:
( ) No difficulty ( ) Age appropriate ( ) Slurred ( ) Aphasic ( ) Deficit

Gastrointestinal:
Frequency:_____ Last BM:_____
( ) Change in bowel habits ( ) Constipation ( ) Diarrhea ( ) Nausea
( ) Vomiting ( ) +Bowel sounds ( ) −Bowel sounds ( ) Bleeding ( ) Weight
change ( ) Difficulty swallowing ( ) Abdominal distention ( ) Change in
appetite ( ) Hernia

Genitourinary:
Last voiding:_____AM/PM ( ) Change in bladder habits ( ) Burning
( ) Frequency ( ) Retention ( ) Urgency ( ) Incontinence ( ) Hematuria ( ) Odor

Neurological:
( ) Alert ( ) Irritable ( ) Lethargic ( ) Comatose ( ) MAE ( ) Hand grasp
( ) Pearl
Infant—Cry: ( ) Strong ( ) Weak
 Fontanel: ( ) Flat ( ) Sunken ( ) Bulging
 Suck: ( ) Strong ( )Weak
Child—Oriented: ( ) Person ( ) Place ( ) Time

Appearance/Behavior:
( ) Appropriate ( ) Flat ( ) Agitated ( ) Frightened ( ) Shy

Growth/Development:
( ) Age-appropriate milestones ( ) Delayed

Musculoskeletal:
( ) Developmental milestones met ( ) Fractures ( ) Weakness ( ) Change in mobility

Integumentary:
( ) Intact ( ) Lacerations ( ) Discolorations ( ) Rash ( ) Dry ( ) Cool ( ) Warm
( ) Diaphoretic ( ) Burns ( ) Bruises ( ) Excoriation ( ) Abrasions ( ) Rash
( ) Jaundice

Reproductive:
( ) Vaginal tag ( ) Undescended testes ( ) Hypospadius

Note: Comments can be added to any component of this assessment. After completion of the infant's assessment, the infant's plan of care was designed.

Outcome Standards

1. The infant admission assessment is accurate and complete.
2. The infant's plan of care was designed by nurse doing the assessment and reflects the assessment of the infant.
3. The infant's assessment and plan of care were completed within __ hours of the infant's admission.*
4. Within __ hours after the child's admission, the parents verbalized an orientation to the clinical unit.*

*The time period required for completion of the infant's assessment and plan of care is defined by hospital policy.

The next unit of care combines the growth and development standards with the care needed by an adolescent who has tried to commit suicide. It is essential that these standards are combined, because the interventions for a child in another stage of growth and development are not the same as those for an adolescent.

POTENTIAL SUICIDE—ADOLESCENT

Goals

1. The patient's environment will be free of further harm or the potential of another suicide attempt.
2. The patient and parent will verbalize concerns, fears, and needs surrounding the suicide attempt.

3. The parents will verbalize an understanding of the recommendations resulting from psychological evaluation.
4. The parents will verbalize an understanding of the contribution of psychological evaluation to prevention of suicide.
5. The patient will remain free of harm while in the hospital.
6. The patient will express concern over self or expressions which reflect goals or events.
7. The patient and parents will express their emotional distress.
8. The parents will interact positively with their child, with support from staff.
9. The parents will assume responsibility for the patient's safety needs.

Process Standards

On admission:

1. Place on constant observation until psychological evaluation can be performed.
2. Place in room near nurse's station so assistance can be provided quickly if employee watching child requests help. Remove all unnecessary objects from room.
3. Dress patient in pajamas and remove clothing from room.
4. Search all personal belongings brought into the room.
5. Notify security that a high-risk patient is on the unit.
6. Identify method used for suicide attempt.
7. Question child regarding thoughts about future attempts:
   a. Is a plan set?
   b. What is it?
   c. Is it feasible?
   d. Does the teen have access to methodology?
   e. What is the time frame?

   Ensure child does not have access to plan.
8. Evaluate history for recent losses or low self-esteem.
9. Be clear about unit expectations (unit boundaries, etc.).
10. Determine visiting privileges according to the physician and parent/guardian comments.

11. Determine telephone privileges according to the physician and parent/guardian.
12. Meet immediate physical needs and evaluate system that has been jeopardized.

After admission:

1. Establish supportive environment to foster positive coping and behaviors:
   a. Provide a consistent, stable, limited environment.
   b. Remain calm; be accepting and supportive. Do not act alarmed, make judgments, or place blame. Express "I care" statements and concern for the patient's well-being.
   c. Be clear about your expectations of the patient.
   d. Maintain visiting/telephone privileges.
   e. Offer choices when available.
   f. Keep recreational activities at bedside along with personal hygiene articles and call bell.
   g. Encourage good hygiene and assist in styling hair, makeup, etc.
2. Encourage patient to talk about recent changes and permit feelings of anger, frustration, and fear.
3. Note patient's general behavior (appropriate attention-seeking, destructive, hyperactive, nightmares, poor sleeper, poor eater).
4. Assist parents in being a positive team that cares enough about the child to prevent harmful behavior.
5. Encourage use of community resources that can be supportive to patient and family, such as clergy, friends, etc.

Outcome Standards

At all times:

1. The patient's environment is free of further harm or the potential for another suicide attempt.
2. The patient remains free of harm while in the hospital.
3. The patient expresses concern over self or expressions that reflect goals or events.
4. The patient and parents verbalize their emotional distress.
5. The parents interact positively with their child, with support from staff, as needed.

Before discharge:

1. The parents assume responsibility for the patient's safety needs.
2. The patient and parents verbalize concerns, fears, and needs surrounding suicide attempt.
3. The parents verbalize an understanding of the recommendations resulting from psychological evaluation.
4. The parents verbalize an understanding of the contribution of psychological evaluation to prevention of suicide.

Children in different stages of growth and development respond diiferently to pain. This response and the interventions are related to each child's stage of growth and development. The standards in this unit of care are a combination of the standards related to the care of the toddler and the standards for the care of the child in pain.

PAIN—OLDER TODDLER/PRESCHOOLER

Goals

1. The child will be kept comfortable as possible.
2. The child's parents will be assisted in implementing comforting techniques.

Process Standards

1. Evaluate physical findings indicating pain:
   a. Self-imposed limitation of activity
   b. Clenching teeth and fist
   c. Rigid position
   d. Irritability
   e. Aggression or verbal attack
2. Monitor trends in vital signs, noting tachycardia, tachypnea, and hypertension.
3. Administer analgesics as prescribed and note their effects.

   Note: Post-op status or tissue damage requires continuous pain administration prior to the onset of obvious/severe pain.
4. Explain all procedures to be performed, and encourage child to ask questions. Tell child what he or she will see, feel, hear, etc.

5. Encourage parents to remain with child and offer soothing techniques.
   a. Hold
   b. Rock
   c. Speak softly
   d. Touch
6. Keep comfort items with child.
7. Use distraction techniques, and encourage parents to continue in your absence from room.
8. Promote restful environment:
   a. Combine nursing procedures to allow for uninterrupted rest periods.
   b. Provide quiet environment, dim lights. Encourage parents to keep familiar items at the bedside (blanket, stuffed animal).
   c. Encourage parents to stay with preschool children.
9. Reinforce that child is not to blame for this pain; he did nothing wrong and pain is not punishment.

Outcome Standards

1. At all times the child is kept comfortable as possible.
2. Within 24 hours the child's parents express that they can use comforting techniques.

The following units of care do not contain interventions that are specific for one stage of growth and development. When these units of care are placed on the child's plan of care, a unit of care related to the growth and developmental stage of the child will need to be added.

REACTIVE AIRWAY DISEASE—ACUTE STABILIZATION PHASE

Goals

1. The child's airways will remain patent.
2. The child will be able to breathe more easily.
3. The child will be well hydrated.

Process Standards

1. Provide respiratory assessment q2h.
2. Monitor trends in vital signs qh. Report deterioration. Maintain on continuous pulse oximeter and A/B monitor.
3. Monitor child's respiratory status closely (q2h).
   a. Observe for respiratory fatigue; if present, notify physician STAT. Have ventilator at bedside along with intubation equipment.
   b. Continuously observe child while in acute distress and encourage parents to remain at the bedside if they reduce child's anxiety.
4. Position patient in 30 to 90-degree Fowler's position or allow to maintain position of comfort.
5. If child is on home bronchodilator, obtain baseline blood level.
6. Provide for uninterrupted rest between treatments.
7. Record effect of treatments.
8. Administer humidified oxygen by mask, nasal cannula, hood, or tent as ordered.
9. Provide continuous pulse oximeter monitoring. Notify physician of oxygen saturation < 90% if it is continuously decreasing and can't be resolved with current plan and orders.
10. Administer inhalation treatment as ordered. Note effects of each treatment. If the condition deteriorates prior to next scheduled treatment, notify physician:
    a. Cyanosis
    b. Decreased air entry
    c. Increased or decreased respiratory rate
    d. Increase in frequency of coughing spasms
    e. Increased restlessness
    f. Lethargy
11. Obtain ABGs and monitor results, reporting abnormal values to the physician during the shift.
12. Establish IV access. Use largest bore catheter possible. Evaluate need for two accesses.
13. Explain all procedures to parents/patient in terms they can understand.
14. Record parent/patient's responses to teaching.

Outcome Standards

At all times:

1. The child's airways are patent.*
2. The child is able to breathe more effectively as indicated by:*
   a. Clear breath sounds
   b. Blood gas values within normal limits
   c. Ease in breathing
3. The child is well hydrated.*

*If not , the physician was notified.

REACTIVE AIRWAY DISEASE—CONVALESCENT PHASE

Goals

1. The child's airways will be patent.
2. The child will be able to breathe more effectively.
3. The child will be able to do his usual activities without dyspnea or fatigue.
4. The child will be well hydrated.
5. The child will not experience a respiratory infection.

Process Standards

1. Auscultate breath sounds and monitor respiratory rate and effort q4h.
2. Administer oxygen therapy as ordered and observe the patient's responses.
3. Provide continuous A/B monitoring:
   a. With IV theophylline
   b. If child is unstable
   c. As ordered
4. Provide continuous pulse oximetry monitoring until stable, with no acute distress X 12, then q shift. Notify physician of deterioration.
5. Allow child to assume position of greatest comfort, keeping head slightly elevated.

6. Observe the patient's response to nebulized bronchodilators as ordered.
7. If on aminophylline therapy, monitor serum levels as ordered and report any level < 10 or > 20.
8. Ensure adequate hydration and evaluate:
   a. Output > 2cc/kg
   b. Sp. Gravity 1.003–1.020 (as ordered)
   c. Moist mucous membranes
   d. Good skin turgor
9. Weigh daily.
10. Maintain calm environment.
11. Explain all procedures to parents/patient in terms they can understand.
12. Record parents'/patient's responses to teaching.

Outcome Standards

At all times:

1. The child's airways are patent.*
2. The child is able to breathe more effectively as indicated by:*
   a. Clear breath sounds
   b. Blood gas values within normal limits
   c. Increasing ease in breathing
   d. Color of skin indicating adequate oxygenation
   e. Decreased anxiety
3. The child can do his usual activities without dyspnea or fatigue.*
4. The child is well hydrated.*
5. The child is not experiencing a respiratory infection:*
   a. Breath sounds clear
   b. Sputum clear
   c. Temperature within normal limits

*If not, the physician was notified.

REACTIVE AIRWAY DISEASE—PARENT TEACHING

Goals

1. The child and parents identify factors that precipitate attacks and how they intend to decrease their frequency.
2. The parents identify when they will need to seek assistance of health care personnel.
3. The parents verbalize a clear understanding of the medication regime.
4. The child and his parents understand the importance of balancing exercise and rest.

Process Standards

1. Teach the patient/parent to avoid contact with others who have upper respiratory infections.
2. Assist the patient/parent to identify precipitating factors that led to the attack that caused this admission.
3. Instruct the patient/parent on how to minimize contact with irritants at home and/or school (smoke, dust, pollen).
4. Teach the patient/parent about the reason for and use of prescribed medications. Review their side effects and caution against the use of over-the-counter drugs. School nurses will need to be aware of the child's medication regime.
5. Reinforce the benefits of physical exercise but stress the importance of rest and not overexerting to the point of fatigue.
6. Encourage questions and allow parents to vent concerns and feelings.
7. Instruct parents on when they should seek health care assistance (change in normal behavior, mild attacks becoming more frequent, chronic cough, shortness of breath, or pallor).
8. Record parents'/patient's responses to teaching.

Outcomes

Within forty-eight hours of admission:

1. The child and parents can identify factors that precipitate attacks and how they intend to decrease their frequency.

2. The parents can identify when they will need to seek assistance of health care personnel.
3. The parents verbalize a clear understanding of the medication regime.
4. The child and his parents verbalize the importance of balancing exercise and rest.

SUMMARY

The purpose of this section was to illustrate how standards of growth and development can be written. The standards can be included with other standards in a unit of care. Or you can develop a unit of care for each stage of growth and development. Because there are units of care like *Reactive Airway Disease* that are appropriate for care of children in more than one stage of growth and development, it is useful to have both types of units of care.

You have completed the section "Writing Standards for the Care of Children."

SECTION 2

Writing Standards
for Perioperative Care

Standards are needed to define the care of the patient as he proceeds through the phases of perioperative care. His plan of care begins at preoperative assessment and ends on discharge from the Postanesthesia Care Unit. If the patient is being discharged the same day as his surgery, the assessment related to his needs at home and the teaching needed to ensure a smooth postoperative recovery also should be included in the unit of care. The rationale for combining the standards from all the perioperative areas on the patient's plan of care is to prevent fragmentation and to increase the efficiency of the delivery of care.

In some surgical areas the units of care for the perioperative clinical areas have been written for each of the areas and kept separately. For example, the Preoperative Assessment is separated from the Operative and Postanesthesia Assessments in the patient's record. Thus, the clinicians are not able to easily compare their assessments to the baseline assessments made preoperatively.

The same is true for the process and outcome standards. If the patient is experiencing health problems preoperatively that affect the care he needs in the operative and postanesthesia phases of his surgery and the clinicians do not have easy access to this information, the patient's needs may not be met, resulting in negative outcomes. Thus, writing the standards for each of the perioperative phases *without* combining them as a unit of care can result in negative patient outcomes while implementing the perioperative care.

Because the patient usually moves rapidly from one phase of perioperative care to another, perioperative units of care should include the care from preoperative through postanesthesia care. The process and content standards for the perioperative periods define:

1. Preoperative period
   a. Assessment
   b. Interventions and observations
   c. Teaching
   d. Evaluation of patient outcomes

2. Operative period
   a. Assessment
   b. Interventions and observations
   c. Evaluation of patient outcomes

3. Postanesthesia period
   a. Assessment
   b. Interventions and observations
   c. Evaluation of patient outcomes

The format for this section is designed to assist you to write standards for the perioperative care of patients, i.e.,

1. Common needs of patients preoperatively
2. Needs of patients preoperatively related to the patients' specific health problems, care needs, or nursing diagnoses
3. Common needs of patients intraoperatively
4. Standards related to a specific surgical procedure
5. Common needs of patients in the Postanesthesia Care Unit
6. Needs of patients immediately postoperatively related to the surgical procedure
7. Needs of patients in Same-day Surgery

PREOPERATIVE PERIOD

The standards for the preoperative period include the preoperative preparation, preoperative teaching, and the baseline assessment of the patient.

Goals

1. The patient will understand:
   a. The care during each of the perioperative phases and the patient's participation
   b. Postoperative care
   c. Care required after discharge
   d. Community agencies that might be needed to assist the patient
2. The patient will be prepared for surgery:
   a. Physically
   b. Psychologically
3. The patient's family will understand:
   a. What the patient will be doing during each of the perioperative phases
   b. Their role in being supportive to the patient
4. The patient's baseline assessment will be accurate, pertinent, and documented.
5. The patient's valuables will remain safe throughout the perioperative period.
6. The patient's record will be complete before the patient leaves for the operating room.

Process and Content Standards

1. Describe the physical preparation for surgery.
2. Inform patient of visits from hospital personnel.
3. Identify the patient's perception of surgery: misconceptions, previous problems, and postop expectations.
4. Ascertain fears/allergies related to anesthesia for the surgery.
5. Answer the patient's questions.
6. Describe the patient's expected condition after surgery.

7. Explain the care during the operative phase.
   a. Position on the table
   b. Use of the monitor
   c. Draping
   d. IV administration
   e. Transfer to the recovery room

8. Explain the care during the recovery phase.
   a. Oxygen by nasal prongs
   b. Monitoring vital signs
   c. Coughing, deep breathing, leg exercises
   d. Pain relief
   e. Notification of family
   f. Length of stay

9. Explain/demonstrate postop activities—return demonstration by patient.
   a. Turning in bed
   b. Deep breathing and coughing
   c. Splint incision
   d. Moving legs
   e. Dorsiflexion and plantar flexion of the feet
   f. Range of motion exercises
   g. Activities for specific surgery

10. Remove makeup, nail polish, hair pins, and jewelry.
11. Provide clothing required for the operating room prior to surgery.
12. Surgical shave prep, if ordered.
13. Ask patient if his bowels moved within the last twenty-four hours. Provide laxative/enema PRN (as ordered).
14. Complete the preoperative checklist. Examples of items:[1]
    a. Consent for surgery signed
    b. History and physical charted
    c. Lab results obtained for tests ordered
    d. Preop medication given, and time

15. Explain examinations and lab tests.
16. If the patient's anxiety and fear continue to increase before surgery, notify the physician.

17. Ascertain if the patient will be wearing a prosthesis or hearing aid to surgery.
18. Ask the patient if he has loose teeth, dentures, or capped teeth.
19. Provide a safe place for valuables, contact lenses, prostheses, and ambulation aids.
20. Explain the surgical routine and postoperative care to the family. Answer their questions:
    a. Preop holding area
    b. Visiting hours
    c. Surgical waiting room during recuperation
    d. Helping the patient during recuperation
21. After assessment of the patient, create his plan of care.[2] Include:
    a. Allergies
    b. Condition of teeth
    c. Blood ordered and number of units available
    d. Level of anxiety and whether surgeon notified if it is increasing
    e. Abnormal results from tests
    f. Patient health problems that can be exacerbated during the perioperative period. Some examples are:[3]
       1. Back pain, arryhthmias, seizures, arthritis
       2. Ability to see and hear
       3. Medications such as: heparin, insulin, steroids, antihypertensive agents, and antidepressive drugs
       4. Abnormal lab values: low red blood count, elevated white count, low thrombocyte count

Two examples of standards related to planning and implementing care related to patient health problems are found after the outcome standards for the preoperative period.

Outcome Standards

Before surgery:

1. The patient can explain:
   a. The care during each of the perioperative phases and the patient's participation
   b. Postoperative care
   c. Care required after discharge

    d. Community agencies that might be needed to assist the patient

2. The patient can demonstrate:
   a. Coughing and deep breathing
   b. Turning
   c. Leg exercises
   d. Incentive spirometer

3. Before the patient leaves for surgery:
   a. All items on the preoperative checklist are completed and documented.
   b. The patient's baseline assessment is accurate, pertinent, and documented.
   c. The patient's plan of care is accurate and pertinent.

4. The patient's family members can explain:
   a. What the patient will be doing during each of the perioperative phases
   b. Their role in being supportive to the patient

5. During the preoperative phase there is an absence of moderate anxiety or panic. If symptoms related to these problems occur, they are reported immediately to the physician.

An example of a *medical diagnosis* that affects the perioperative care is as follows.

DIABETES MELLITUS

Preoperative Period
Goals

1. Pertinent data concerning the patient's medical diagnosis will be recorded and reported to the surgeon before he leaves for the operating room.
2. The patient will be wearing a bracelet with pertinent information concerning his medical diagnosis before the patient leaves for the operating room.

Process Standards

1. Document on patient's plan of care:
   a. Results of blood glucose testing and when last tested
   b. Results of urine testing and when last tested
   c. Significant results reported to the surgeon
2. Report significant results to the surgeon before the patient leaves for the operating room.
3. Place a bracelet containing pertinent information about the patient's medical condition on the patient's arm before he leaves for the operating room.

Outcome Standards

Before the patient leaves for the operating room:

1. The following data are listed on the patient's plan of care:
   a. Results of blood glucose testing and when last tested
   b. Results of urine testing and when last tested
   c. Significant results reported to the surgeon
2. Significant results related to testing the patient's blood or urine for glucose were reported to the surgeon.
3. A bracelet containing pertinent information about the patient's medical condition was placed on his arm.

Intraoperative Period
Goal

1. The patient will not experience hypoglycemia or ketoacidosis during the intraoperative period.

Process Standards

1. Read the information on the patient's bracelet or the preop care plan regarding his medical condition.
2. Inform the surgeon and anesthetist concerning the patient's medical condition.
3. Observe continuously for changes in the patient's health status indicating hypoglycemia or ketoacidosis.

Outcome Standard

1. During the intraoperative period, the patient did not experience hypoglycemia or ketoacidosis.

Postanesthesia Period
Goal

1. The patient will not experience hypoglycemia or ketoacidosis during the postanesthesia period.

Process Standards

1. Read the information on the patient's bracelet or the preop care plan regarding his medical condition.
2. Observe continuously for changes in the patient's health status indicating hypoglycemia or ketoacidosis.
3. Inform the surgeon concerning significant changes in the patient's condition.

Outcome Standards

1. During the postanesthesia period, the patient did not experience hypoglycemia or ketoacidosis.
2. At all times, significant changes in the patient's condition were reported to the surgeon and anesthesiologist.

An example of medications the patient is receiving that might affect the care in the perioperative period is the

ADMINISTRATION OF ANTICOAGULANTS[4]

Preoperative Period
Goals

1. Pertinent data related to the medications administered to the patient will be recorded and reported to the surgeon before the patient leaves for the operating room.
2. The patient will be wearing a bracelet with pertinent information concerning his medical diagnosis before the patient leaves for the operating room.

Process Standards

1. Document on the patient's plan of care the time the last dose of heparin or coumadin was administered to the patient.
2. Place a bracelet containing pertinent information about the patient's medication on the patient's arm before he leaves for the operating room.

Outcome Standards

Before the patient leaves for the operating room:

1. The time the last dose of heparin or coumadin was administered to the patient was documented on the patient's plan of care.
2. A bracelet containing pertinent information about the patient's medication was placed on the patient's arm.

Intraoperative Period
Goal

1. The patient will not experience hemorrhage during the intraoperative period.

Process Standards

1. Read the information on the patient's bracelet or the preop care plan regarding his medication.
2. Inform the surgeon and anesthetist concerning the patient's medication.
3. Observe for excessive bleeding continuously.

Outcome Standard

1. During the intraoperative period, the patient did not experience hemorrhage.

Postanesthesia Period
Goal

1. The patient will not experience hemorrhage during the postanesthesia period.

Process Standards

1. Read the information on the patient's bracelet or the preop care plan regarding his medication.
2. Observe continuously for excessive bleeding.
3. Inform the surgeon concerning any significant bleeding.

Outcome Standards

1. During the postanesthesia period, the patient did not experience hemorrhage.
2. At all times, significant bleeding was reported to the surgeon.

CARE DURING THE INTRAOPERATIVE PERIOD

The overall goal of the care of patients during the intraoperative period is prevention of injury to the patient. The process and content standards written for this period include:

1. Commonalities in care during the operative period
2. Specific surgical procedures
3. Needs of patients during the intraoperative period

The following units of care are examples of care implemented during the intraoperative period:

1. Needs of patients identified during Preoperative Assessment of the patient:
   a. Back pain
   b. Recently taken medications such as anticoagulants, mellaril

2. Commonly implemented procedures:
   a. Use of the electrosurgical unit during surgery
   b. Sponges, sharps, and instrument counts
   c. Transfer of the patient from stretcher to the operating table

3. Standards related to specific surgical procedures:
   a. Preparation of the skin
   b. Position of the patient
   c. Care of organs to be implanted or transplanted
   d. Care of specimens
   e. Medications/infusions to be administered during surgery

    f. Lab reports/X-rays available during surgery

4. The psychologic care of the patient when awake:
   a. In the holding area
   b. In surgery—local or regional anesthesia

5. Maintaining the security of the personal articles brought to the operating room:
   a. Valuables
   b. Hearing aid
   c. Prosthesis

Goals

1. The patient will not experience any injuries.
2. The patient will not experience preventable complications.
3. The patient will not experience an infection.
4. The patient's valuables will remain safe.
5. The patient's anxiety will not escalate.
6. Organs for transplantation will remain safe and viable.
7. Specimens will be in good condition upon entry into the laboratory.

Process Standards

The following process standards are implemented for *all* patients who require surgery. These standards are added to the standards for specific surgical procedures to create units of care for the surgical unit of care.

1. Correctly identify the patient.
2. In the holding area, observe the patient continuously for changes in health status.
3. Implement aseptic technique throughout the surgical procedure.
4. Maintain the patient's privacy.
5. Prepare the patient's skin according to the:
   a. Type of surgery
   b. Surgeon's orders

6. Position the patient in relation to:
   a. Type of surgery
   b. Surgeon's orders
   c. Safety of the patient's body during surgery

7. Monitor the patient during surgery:
   a. Level of oxygenation
   b. Cardiovascular function
   c. Changes in the level of consciousness
   d. Changes in the patient's behavior when awake
   e. Fluid intake and blood loss

Outcome Standards

1. Throughout the intraoperative period the patient experienced:
   a. No injuries
   b. No preventable complications
2. When awake, the patient's anxiety did not escalate during the intraoperative period.
3. Organs for transplantation remained safe and viable.
4. Specimens obtained during surgery reached the laboratory in satisfactory condition.
5. Patient's X-rays, lab reports were available as needed.
6. Specimen bottles were labeled correctly; they were taken to the pathology lab.

PROCEDURES

The following are examples of procedures commonly used in the intraoperative period.

Use of Electro Surgical Unit During Surgery

Goal

1. The patient's skin will not be burned during surgery.

Process Standards

1. Before the surgery:
   a. A grounding pad will be properly placed and attached to machine with appropriate adapter.
   b. Bovie cord will be properly connected.
2. Observe bovie output and monitor change as necessary.

Outcome Standards

1. At the end of the procedure the patient's skin is intact and not burned.[5]

Sponges, Sharps and Instrument Counts[6]

Goal

1. The patient will be protected from sponges, instruments, and sharps being left in his body cavity during surgery.

Process Standards

1. Count all sponges, sharps, and instruments:
   a. At the beginning of each case
   b. Before each body cavity or organ is closed
   c. Before skin is closed
   d. At the completion of the case
   e. At any change of personnel
2. Record counts on work sheet. Add all sponges, sharps, or instruments added to the field during the case to the work sheet.
3. All counts will be done by both the scrub nurse and the circulating nurse together.
4. No trash or instruments will leave the room until a correct sponge count has been obtained.

Outcome Standards

1. All sponges, sharps, and instruments are counted:
   a. At the beginning of each case
   b. Before each body cavity or organ is closed
   c. Before skin is closed
   d. At the completion of the case
   e. At any change of personnel
2. All sponges, sharps, and instrument counts are recorded.

Transfer of Patient from Stretcher/Bed to the Operating Table[7]

Goals

1. The patient will have no alteration in integrity of any invasive lines, tubes, or leads.
2. The patient's body alignment will be optimal.
3. The patient will receive no injury during transfer.

Process Standards

1. Lock bed or stretcher.
2. Lock operating room table.
3. Make sure bed, stretcher, and operating room table are the same height.
4. Observe that all invasive lines, tubes, leads, etc., are intact and functioning properly.
5. Make sure two people are in attendance during transfer.
6. Make sure the patient is always attended while on operating room table.
7. Observe patient's position on operating room table and align properly.
8. Place safety strap over patient.
9. Record data concerning transfer on operating room note.

Outcome Standards

Before transfer from stretcher/bed to operating room table and back to stretcher:

1. Bed or stretcher is locked.
2. Operating room table is locked.
3. Bed/stretcher and operating room table are the same height.
4. Two operating room personnel are assisting with transfer.
5. At all times, while on the operating room table, the patient is attended by operating room personnel.
6. At all times during the transfer the integrity of tubes, invasive lines, or leads are maintained.
7. At all times during the transfer the patient is not injured.
8. After the transfer, appropriate data are recorded on the patient's record.

STANDARDS RELATED TO SPECIFIC PROCEDURES

There are standards related to specific surgical procedures and surgeon's preferences that need to be added to the intraoperative standards when patients are experiencing these surgical procedures.

Operative Procedure: Dilatation and Curettage
Goals

1. The patient will not experience lumbosacral strain postoperatively.
2. The patient will not experience disturbances caused by rapid alterations in venous return.

Process Standards

1. Make sure stirrups are well padded.
2. Lift both legs at the same time when putting the legs in stirrups.
3. Raise and lower legs slowly when positioning the patient.

Outcome Standards

1. Postoperatively, the patient is not experiencing lumbosacral strain.
2. The patient did not experience changes in vital signs after positioning in the operating room and after transferring the patient to the postanesthesia care unit.

Operative Procedure: Carotid Endarterectomy[8]
Goals

1. The patient will not experience decreased blood flow to the carotid vertebral artery system.
2. The amount of the patient's irrigation fluid instilled and irrigation drainage will be accurately monitored and recorded.

Process Standards

1. The patient's position is supine, with head slightly extended toward the opposite side (to prevent excessive rotation of the head and extension of the neck).
2. Monitor and record the amount of irrigation fluid instilled and irrigation drainage.

3. Before surgery begins, check preop documentation to identify if
   a. Blood is available as ordered
   b. The patient's X-ray film

Operative Procedure: Some Orthopedic Surgeries
Use of a Tourniquet During Surgery[9]
Goals

1. The patient will not experience trauma to viable tissues.
2. The effect of the tourniquet on the patient's limb will be optimal for the surgery.

Process Standards

1. Place tourniquet as high on the extremity as possible.
2. Make sure tourniquet ends overlap at least 2 inches.
3. Do not allow solutions for preparation to pool under the tourniquet.
4. If surgery is being performed on an upper extremity, do not apply tourniquet at the elbow.
5. Tourniquet pressure as ordered by the surgeon.
6. Monitor tourniquet time and setting q10 minutes.
7. Release tourniquet after 2 hours.

Outcome Standards

1. During the surgery there was no excessive bleeding in the wound.
2. Before leaving the operating room:
   a. The tourniquet was released.
   b. There was not visible damage to viable tissues.

POSTANESTHESIA CARE

Goals

1. The patient will have a patent airway.
2. The patient will not experience preventable complications.
3. The patient's pain will be controlled.
4. The patient's valuables will remain safe throughout the perioperative period.

5. The patient will be awake before discharge from the postanesthesia care unit.

6. The patient's condition will be stable before discharge.

Process Standards

1. Position patient to maintain patent airway at all times.
2. Initiate oxygen.
3. Monitor effectiveness of airway support.
4. Initiate PACU record and scoring system on admission.
5. Vital signs on admission, q15 minutes, and PRN:
   a. Blood pressure
   b. Pulse
   c. Respirations
6. Provide safety measures:
   a. Siderails up
   b. Apply soft restraint, as appropriate
   c. Apply bumper pads, as appropriate
   d. Wheels locked on stretcher
7. Assess on admission and q__minutes
   a. Cardiovascular parameters
   b. Respiratory parameters
   c. Invasive lines and sites as appropriate
   d. Gastro-intestinal parameters
   e. Pulse oximetry
   f. Patient temperature
   g. Dressings/operative site(s)
   h. Drains and tubes
   i. Intake and output
   j. Neurovascular signs
   k. Regional block reversal

Notify physician of significant alterations in any of the asssessments.

8. Medicate per physician order. If medication is ineffective, notify physician.
9. Provide emotional support.

10. Connect tubes to drainage systems. Ensure drainage systems are functioning effectively.
11. Encourage coughing and deep breathing PRN as appropriate.
12. Assist in changing positions as needed.
13. Check physician's orders and implement accordingly.
14. Discharge from PACU after patient meets PACU Scoring System or with Department of Anesthesia approval.
15. Transfer to clinical unit.

Outcome Standards

At all times:

1. The patient's airway is patent.
2. The patient is not experiencing preventable complications.
3. The patient's pain is controlled.
4. The patient's condition is stable before discharge:
   a. Vital signs are stable and within expected limits.
   b. Hemodynamic parameters are stable and within expected limits.
   c. Approval obtained from the Department of Anesthesia and/or expected discharge score on the PACU Scoring System.

When the patient is admitted, has surgery, and is discharged the same day, there are standards for additional components to be added to each perioperative unit of care. These are:

1. Admission to the Same-day Surgery Unit
2. Postanesthesia care until discharge
3. Post-discharge phone call

ADMISSION TO THE SAME-DAY SURGERY UNIT

Goals

The *goals* are the same as preoperative care for all surgery. There are two additional *goals*:

1. The patient will be oriented to his room and procedures of the Same-day Surgical Unit.

2. The patient and/or family will be able to explain the care of the patient at home.

Process Standards

1. Check unit for readiness:
   a. Bed completed
   b. Stand stocked with patient-comfort items
   c. All equipment working
2. When patient arrives, greet patient by name and introduce self.
3. Apply and/or check ID band and confirm accuracy.
4. Check vital signs.
5. Inquire if patient has had or has any recent symptoms of cold or flu. If so, notify physician.
6. N.P.O. since _____.
7. Inform patient of location of bed, bathroom, locker, and fire doors.
8. Instruct patient on location and use of bed control as appropriate, nurse call light, TV controls if available, telephone, bathroom-assist light.
9. Complete Patient Belongings and Valuables Record.
10. Apply allergy band on patient and identify drug sensitivities where and when appropriate.
11. Observe patient and family involvement in plan of care and encourage their participation.
12. Check physician orders and carry out accordingly.
13. Monitor lab results.
14. Review chart content and assembly.
15. Initiate preoperative checklist.[10]
16. Surgical prep as ordered.
17. IV started: _____
    with _____ in _____
    at _____ by _____
18. Transfer to surgery/holding room via _____
    at _____.

Outcome Standards

The *outcomes* are the same as preoperative care for all surgery. There are two additional *outcomes*.

Before the patient leaves for the Operating Room:

1. The patient verbalizes an orientation to his room and procedures of the Same-day Surgical Unit.
2. The patient and/or family can explain the care of the patient at home.

SAME-DAY SURGERY UNIT— POSTANESTHESIA CARE UNTIL DISCHARGE[11]

Goals

1. The patient's health status will be assessed until he can safely be discharged from the hospital.
2. The patient and/or family will understand the care of the patient on discharge.
3. The patient and/or family will understand how to obtain resources in the community after discharge.

Process Standards

1. Position patient for maximum chest expansion.
2. Check vital signs.
3. Evaluate patient's level of consciousness q15 minutes.
4. Medicate per physician order. If ineffective, report to the physician.
5. Encourage the patient to cough and deep breathe q15 minutes.
6. Encourage the patient to move legs and feet frequently.
7. Observe IV infusion for:
   a. Patency
   b. Rate
   c. Dressing
   d. Phlebitis
8. Observe the surgical site/dressing q15 minutes.

9. When awake, offer the patient small amounts of clear liquids. Observe the patient's tolerance of all intake.
10. Maintain the siderails in the up position until ambulatory.

When the patient is able to ambulate:

11. Assist patient with first ambulation and observe tolerance.
12. Monitor first postop voiding as appropriate.
13. IV discontinued at_____.
14. Notify physician if the patient has:
    a. Abnormalities in vital signs
    b. Abnormalities in respiratory function
    c. Excessive bleeding from incision/surgical site
    d. Persistent nausea and vomiting
15. Discharge patient upon physician order after patient has met Anesthesia Discharge Criteria.

Outcome Standards

Before discharge:

16. The patient and/or family can verbalize:
    a. Care of the patient on discharge
    b. How to obtain resources in the community after discharge
2. The patient's health status meets the criteria for discharge.

POST-DISCHARGE ASSESSMENT[12]

In many hospitals a staff member telephones patients the day after being discharged from Same-day Surgery to assess how they are feeling and if they are experiencing any complications. Listed below are questions commonly asked during the telephone call.

Goals

1. The patient's progress post-discharge will be assessed and recorded.
2. Any problems identified during the phone call to the patient will be referred to the appropriate health professional.

Process Standards

Inquire about the patient's health status, as he describes it.

1. Are you experiencing pain/discomfort?
2. Is your pain medication effective?
3. If you have a dressing, is it dry?
4. Do you have any bleeding, drainage, redness, or swelling?
5. Are you having any trouble urinating?
6. Are you able to tolerate liquids and/or food?
7. Are you experiencing any nausea or vomiting?
8. Are you experiencing any numbness, tingling of your arms or legs?
9. Have you made your follow-up appointment with the physician?
10. Do you have any questions?

As a result of the phone call, the physician is notified if the patient is experiencing complications or is not progressing as planned.

Outcome Standards

11. The patient's progress after discharge was assessed and accurately recorded.
12. New health problems or complications of surgery were reported to the physician within _____ hours.

Now all the components of perioperative care will be assembled in the following example, *Care of the Patient Undergoing Cataract Surgery.*

CARE OF THE PATIENT UNDERGOING CATARACT SURGERY

The perioperative plan of care for the patient undergoing cataract surgery begins with standards for the Preoperative Teaching and ends with the Post-discharge Assessment.

Goals

The goals include the goals for the care to be implemented in all the periods of perioperative care.

Preoperative Teaching

1. The patient will understand:
   a. The care during each of the perioperative phases and the patient's participation
   b. Care required after discharge
      1. How to prevent increasing intraocular pressure
      2. Care of the eye
      3. How to take medications and instill eye drops
   c. Observations that need to be reported to the physician
   d. Community agencies that might be needed to assist the patient
2. The patient's family members will understand:
   a. What the patient will be doing during each of the perioperative phases
   b. Their role in being supportive to the patient

Admission of the Patient and Preoperative Care

1. The patient will be admitted to the Same-day Surgery Unit.
2. The patient will be prepared for surgery:
   a. Physically
   b. Psychologically
3. The patient's baseline assessment will be accurate, and pertinent.
4. The patient will not experience any falls during hospitalization.
5. The patient's valuables will remain safe throughout the perioperative period.

Intraoperative Period

1. The patient will not experience any injuries.
2. The patient will not experience preventable complications.
3. The patient will not experience an infection.
4. The patient's valuables will remain safe throughout the perioperative period.
5. The patient's anxiety will not escalate during the intraoperative period.
6. Organs for transplantation will remain safe and viable.
7. Specimens obtained during surgery will remain safe during surgery and will be sent to the lab.

Postanesthesia Period

1. The patient will have a patent airway.
2. The patient will not experience preventable complications.
3. The patient's pain will be controlled.
4. The patient's valuables will remain safe throughout the perioperative period.
5. The patient will be awake before discharge from the PACU.
6. The patient's condition will be stable before discharge.

Same-day Surgery—Postanesthesia Care until Discharge

1. The patient will be oriented to his room and procedures of the Same-day Surgical unit.
2. The patient will be prepared for discharge on the same day as his surgery.
3. The patient and/or family can explain the care of the patient at home.

Post-discharge Assessment

1. The patient's progress after discharge will be assessed and recorded.
2. Any problems identified during the phone call to the patient will be referred to the appropriate health professional.

The process and content standards will be presented in the order that they will be implemented. The standards will be labeled with the titles of each of the components for clarity.

Preoperative Teaching[13]

The content standards for preoperative teaching are a combination of the general preoperative teaching and those related to the teaching of the patient having cataract surgery.

Teaching is usually done prior to surgery. It may be done in the surgeon's office or on a visit to the hospital before the surgery.

1. Describe the physical preparation for surgery.
2. Identify the patient's perception of surgery: misconceptions, previous problems, and postop expectations.
3. Ascertain fears/allergies related to anesthesia for the surgery.
4. Answer the patient's questions.
5. Describe the patient's expected condition after surgery.
6. Explain the care during the operative phase.
   a. Position on the table

    b. Use of the monitor

    c. Draping

    d. IV administration

    e. Transfer to the recovery room

7. Explain the care during the recovery phase.
   a. Oxygen by nasal prongs
   b. Monitoring vital signs
   c. Pain relief
   d. Notification of family
   e. Length of stay

8. Remove makeup, nail polish, hair pins, and jewelry.

9. Explain examinations and lab tests.

10. Explain the surgical routine and postoperative care to the family and answer their questions:
    a. Preop holding area
    b. Visiting hours
    c. Surgical waiting room during recuperation
    d. How they can help the patient during recuperation

11. Instruct the patient concerning care after discharge:
    a. Prevent increasing intraocular pressure. Examples are: no bending, lifting, straining, coughing, sneezing.
    b. Avoid touching or rubbing the eye.
    c. Avoid constipation.

12. Report to the surgeon:
    a. Sudden, sharp pain in eye
    b. Pain unrelieved by medication
    c. Nausea and vomiting
    d. Halos around lights
    e. Increasing redness in the operative eye
    f. Yellow, foul-smelling drainage
    g. Elevated temperature

13. If patient has implant, report to the surgeon:
    a. Distorted vision
    b. Blurred or cloudy vision

14. Instruct regarding:
    a. Medications
    b. Care of eye
    c. Adjustments to glasses or contacts

Admission of the Patient and Preoperative Care

The process standards for admission to the Same-day Surgery unit: Preoperative care is a combination of the general preoperative care and those related to the care of the patient having cataract surgery in Same-day Surgery.

1. Check unit for readiness:
   a. Bed completed
   b. Stand stocked with patient-comfort items
   c. All equipment working

2. When patient arrives, greet patient by name and introduce self.
3. Apply and/or check ID band and confirm accuracy.
4. Check vital signs.
5. Inquire if patient has had or has any recent symptoms of cold or flu. If so, notify physician.
6. Nothing by mouth—time started
7. Inform patient of location of bed, bathroom, locker, and fire doors.
8. Instruct patient on location and use of bed control as appropriate, nurse call light, TV controls if available, telephone, bathroom-assist light.
9. Complete Patient Belongings and Valuables Record.
10. Apply allergy band on patient and identify drug sensitivities where and when appropriate.
11. Observe patient and family involvement in plan of care and encourage their participation.
12. Check physician orders and carry out accordingly.
13. Monitor lab results.
14. Review chart content and assembly.
15. Initiate preoperative checklist.
16. Provide clothing required for the operating room prior to surgery.
17. Assist the patient with preop preparations as needed.
18. Start IV, infuse solution.

19. Determine method of transfer to surgery/holding room.
20. Monitor patient's anxiety and fear. Notify the surgeon if patient's anxiety is increasing to the moderate or panic level.
21. Ascertain if the patient will be wearing a prosthesis or hearing aid to surgery.
22. Ask the patient if he has loose teeth, dentures, or capped teeth.
23. Assess the ability of the patient to see: Left eye _____ Right eye _____.
24. Observe for coughing and/or retching. Report immediately to the surgeon.
25. Administer the preop medication as ordered.
26. Administer the eye drops as ordered into the conjunctival sac.
27. Assess condition of artificial joints, pacemaker.
28. Assess condition of the teeth—retainers, bridges, plates.
29. Identify who will take patient home—place on plan of care.*
30. Identify who will assist the patient in his home—place on plan of care.*

*If patient requires additional assistance, notify discharge planner.

Intraoperative Period*

The process standards for Same-day Surgery intraoperative care are a combination of the general intraoperative care and those related to the care of the patient having cataract surgery.

1. Correctly identify the patient on arrival to the Holding Area.
2. In the Holding Area, observe the patient continuously for changes in health status. Report significant changes to the surgeon and anesthetist.
3. Review:
   a. Operative permit signed
   b. Allergies to prep solution (identified on the plan of care)
   c. Needs resulting in alteration to the position during surgery
   d. Preop checklist
4. Observe the level of relaxation of the patient before surgery. Report moderate levels of anxiety to the surgeon.
5. Administer eye drops as ordered.

Transfer of the patient to the operating room table:

6. Lock the bed or stretcher.

7. Lock the operating room table.

8. Make sure the bed, stretcher, and operating room table are the same height.

9. Observe that all invasive lines, tubes, leads, etc., are intact and functioning properly.

10. Make sure two people are in attendance during transfer.

11. Observe patient's position on operating room table and align properly.

12. Place safety strap over patient.

13. Make sure the patient is always attended while on the operating room table.

14. Positioning:
    a. The patient is supine. The arm on the operative side may be secured at the patient's side while the other arm is extended on an arm support.
    b. See to additional specification by the surgeon.
    c. See to safety of the patient's body during surgery; modify position according to needs listed on the patient's plan of care.

15. Prepare the patient's skin according to the:
    a. Type of surgery
    b. Additional specification by the surgeon
    c. Safety of the patient in relation to allergies listed on the patient's plan of care

16. Maintain the patient's privacy.

17. Implement aseptic technique throughout the surgical procedure.

18. Avoid extraneous noise.

19. Irrigate eye from inner to outer canthus.

20. Monitor the patient during surgery:
    a. Level of oxygenation
    b. Cardiovascular function
    c. Changes in the level of consciousness
    d. Changes in the patient's behavior when awake
    e. Level of relaxation prior to the removal of the lens

*The standards for the care that will be needed by a specific patient also depend on the type of anesthesia he received.

Postanesthesia Period

The process standards for Same-day Surgery postanesthesia care are a combination of the general postanesthesia care and those related to the care of the patient having cataract surgery.

1. Before the patient arrives, place the bedside stand on unoperative side.
2. Position patient to maintain patent airway at all times.
3. Elevate the patient's head 45 degrees.
4. Initiate oxygen.
5. Monitor effectiveness of airway support.
6. Initiate PACU record and scoring system on admission.
7. Place patient's personal articles, call light, phone, and water within easy reach at all times.
8. Keep side rails up on operative side.
9. Position patient on back or unoperative side.
10. Approach patient from unoperative side.
11. Provide safety measures:
    a. Siderails up
    b. Soft restraint, as appropriate
    c. Bumper pads, as appropriate
    d. Wheels locked on stretcher
12. Assess on admission and q__minutes
    a. Cardiovascular parameters
    b. Respiratory parameters
    c. Invasive lines and sites as appropriate
    d. Gastro-intestinal parameters
    e. Pulse oximetry
    f. Patient temperature
    g. Dressings/operative site(s)
    h. Drains and tubes
    i. Intake and output
    j. Neurovascular signs
    k. Regional block reversal

Notify physician of significant alterations in any of the asssessments.

13. Medicate per physician order. If medication is ineffective, notify physician.

14. Provide emotional support.

15. Assist in changing positions as needed.

16. Check physician's orders and implement accordingly.

17. Discharge from PACU after patient meets PACU Scoring System or with Department of Anesthesia approval.

18. Transfer to clinical unit.

*The standards for the care that will be needed by a specific patient also depend on the type of anesthesia he received.

Same-day Surgery—Postanesthesia Care until Discharge*

The process standards for Same-day Surgery postanesthesia care are a combination of the general postanesthesia care and those related to the care of the patient having cataract surgery.

1. Before the patient arrives, place the bedside stand on unoperative side.

2. Position patient to maintain patent airway at all times.

3. Elevate the patient's head 45 degrees.

4. Maintain the siderails in the up position until ambulatory.

5. Position patient on back or unoperative side.

6. Approach patient from unoperative side.

7. Check vital signs.

8. Evaluate patient's level of consciousness q15 minutes

9. Medicate per physician order. If ineffective, report to the physician.

10. Place patient's personal articles, call light, phone, and water within easy reach *at all times.*

11. Encourage the patient to move his legs and feet frequently.

12. Observe IV infusion for:
    a. Patency
    b. Rate
    c. Dressing
    d. Phlebitis

13. Observe the surgical site/dressing q15 minutes.

14. When patient is awake, offer small amounts of clear liquids. Observe the patient's tolerance of all intake.

When the patient is able to ambulate:[14]

15. Assist patient with first ambulation and observe tolerance.
16. Monitor first postop voiding as appropriate. Assist the patient to the bathroom, unless contraindicated.
17. Discontinue IV at _____.
18. Notify physician of:
    a. Abnormalities in vital signs
    b. Abnormalities in respiratory function
    c. Excessive bleeding from incision/surgical site
    d. Nausea and/or vomiting
19. Reinforce preoperative instruction:
    a. No bending, lifting, straining, coughing, sneezing
    b. Avoid touching or rubbing the eye
20. Report to the surgeon:
    a. Sudden, sharp pain in eye
    b. Pain unrelieved by medication
    c. Nausea and vomiting
    d. Halos around lights
    e. Inflammation
    f. Yellow, foul-smelling drainage
    g. Elevated temperature
21. If patient has an implant, report to the surgeon:
    a. Distorted vision
    b. Blurred or cloudy vision
22. Reinforce preoperative instruction regarding:
    a. Medications
    b. Care of eye
    c. Adjustments to glasses or contacts
23. Ensure patient has someone to drive him home and assist him with his care as needed.
24. Discharge patient upon physician order after patient has met Anesthesia Discharge Criteria.

*The standards for the care that will be needed by a specific patient also depend on the type of anesthesia he received.

Post-discharge Assessment[15]

1. Call the patient after same-day surgery experience.
2. Evaluate patient health status at the time of the inquiry, as appropriate. Suggested questions:
   a. Are you experiencing pain/discomfort? If so, describe _____.
   b. Is your pain medication effective?
   c. Describe the condition of the operative eye. Do you have any bleeding or drainage from either eye?
   d. Are you able to tolerate liquids and/or food?
   e. Are you experiencing any nausea/vomiting?
   f. Are you experiencing any coughing?
   g. Have you read the postoperative instructions?
   h. Explain how you are using your eye drops/ointment.
   i. Do you have any questions?
   j. Have you made your follow-up appointment with your physician?
3. Evaluate the patient's answers. If a health problem or patient care need is present, instruct the patient to call the physician.
4. Provide the patient with a copy of homegoing instructions completed with the surgeon's preferences.

HOMEGOING INSTRUCTIONS

Dear _____,

You recently received cataract surgery in the Same-day Surgery unit at our hospital. As discussed with you after your surgery, you will need to follow certain procedures to continue the healing of your eye.

Care of the Eyes

1. Do not rub your eyes or touch them unless you are putting medication into them or cleaning them.
2. Wash your hands before touching your eyes.
3. Wipe gently around the ____ eye twice daily to remove secretions.
4. Put ____ drops of _____ into the ____ eye ____ times a day.
5. Put ____ amount of _____ ointment into the ____ eye ____ times a day.

Note: Eye drops or ointment should be placed in the space formed when the skin below the lower lid is gently drawn down. DO NOT PLACE ANY MEDICATION DIRECTLY ON THE EYE.

6. When using eye drops or ointment, hold the applicator near the eye, but do not touch eyelids or lashes. Place the heel of the hand holding the eye medication against the face for support.

7. Close the eyes for 1 to 2 minutes after the medication has been given.

8. Gently remove the excess medication with a gauze pad or a cotton ball.

9. Use a separate gauze pad or cotton ball for each eye.

Activity List

Activities*	Date when you can begin:
_____ Driving	_____
_____ Stairs	_____
_____ Walking	_____
_____ Lifting	until approval from surgeon
_____ Bending	until approval from surgeon
_____ Housework	until approval from surgeon
_____ Pushing/Pulling	until approval from surgeon
_____ Shower	
_____ Tub/bath	
_____ Sexual activity	until approval from surgeon

*The items RESTRICTED in the activity list have been specified by your surgeon.

You should avoid straining, coughing, sneezing, and/or vomiting, to prevent injury to the healing eye.

Your surgeon wants you to call if you have any of the following symptoms:

1. Sudden, sharp pain in eye
2. Pain unrelieved by medication
3. Nausea and vomiting
4. Halos around lights
5. Reddened eye
6. Yellow, foul-smelling drainage
7. Elevated temperature

8. Constant cough
9. Frequent sneezing

Your surgeon's phone number is _____.

If you have received an implant, report the following symptoms to the surgeon:

1. Distorted vision
2. Blurred or cloudy vision

Your next appointment with Dr. _____ is _____.

If you have any questions about your progress or activities you can do while you are recovering from surgery, call this number: _____.

Sincerely,

Outcome Standards

All the outcomes for this example will be listed in the order of their implementation. Because the outcomes of one period can result in the modification of or different interventions in ensuing periods, the evaluation of the patient's care in relation to most outcome standards should occur as the patient is being prepared to move to the next perioperative period or at the beginning of the next period. Evaluating the care can prevent such negative outcomes as:

3. The patient required a tourniquet during surgery. The tourniquet was not removed until after there was tissue death. The patient's finger had to be amputated.
4. The patient needed to take his hearing aid to the operating room. It was lost somewhere between the admitting unit and his postoperative unit.
5. The patient had extensive bleeding during surgery, which continued during the postanesthesia period. It was later discovered that the patient had received two injections of an anticoagulant during a diagnostic test shortly before surgery.

If the outcome standards are placed on the patient's plan of care, they can be evaluated as the patient's plan is reviewed *before* the patient is transferred to the next period. Or, the standards can be included on the care plan for the next period which is reviewed at the *beginning* of the next period.

CARE OF THE PATIENT UNDERGOING CATARACT SURGERY

Outcome Standards for Preoperative Teaching

Before surgery:

1. The patient can explain:
   a. The care during each of the perioperative phases and the patient's participation
   b. Postoperative care
      1. Activities
      2. How to take medications
      3. Care of the eye
      4. Symptoms to report to the physician
      5. Prevention of constipation
   c. Community agencies that might be needed to assist the patient

2. The patient can demonstrate:
   a. Coughing and deep breathing
   b. Turning
   c. Leg exercises
   d. Incentive spirometer

3. The patient's family members can explain:
   a. What the patient will be doing during each of the perioperative phases
   b. Their role in being supportive to the patient

Admission of the Patient and Preoperative Care

Before the patient leaves for the operating room:

1. The patient verbalizes an orientation to his room and procedures of the Same-day Surgical Unit.
2. The patient and/or family can explain the care of the patient at home.
3. All items on the preoperative checklist are completed and documented.
4. The patient's baseline assessment is accurate, pertinent, and documented.
5. The patient's plan of care is accurate and pertinent.

6. During the preoperative phase there is an absence of moderate anxiety or panic. If symptoms related to these problems occur, they are reported immediately to the physician.

Intraoperative Period

1. Throughout the intraoperative period the patient experienced:
   a. No injuries
   b. No preventable complications
2. When awake, the patient's anxiety did not escalate during the intraoperative period.
3. Organs for transplantation remained safe and viable.
4. Specimens obtained during surgery reached the laboratory in satisfactory condition.

Postanesthesia Period

At all times:

1. The patient's airway is patent.
2. The patient is not experiencing preventable complications.
3. The patient's pain is controlled.
4. The patient's condition is stable before discharge:
   a. Vital signs stable and within expected limits
   b. Hemodynamic parameters stable and within expected limits
   c. Approval obtained from the Department of Anesthesia and/or expected discharge score on the PACU Scoring System.
5. During the entire perioperative period the patient's valuables were safe.

Same-day Surgery Postanesthesia Care before Discharge:

1. The patient and/or family can verbalize:
   a. The care of the patient on discharge
   b. How to obtain resources in the community after discharge
2. The patient's health status meets the criteria for discharge.

Post-discharge Assessment

1. The patient's progress after discharge was assessed and accurately recorded.

2. New health problems or complications of surgery were reported to the physician within _____ hours.[16]

SUMMARY

When writing standards for the perioperative period, the unit of care for a specific surgical procedure begins during Preoperative Teaching and ends with the patient being transferred to a clinical unit or Post-discharge Assessment. Each of the units of care contain the standards that are common to all patients in each of the perioperative periods as well as those specific for the surgical procedure, anesthesia, and the patient's health problems that affect the care during the perioperative period.

As Chana has stated, "the challenge is to create a care plan that can be individualized for each patient and is not too time consuming for perioperative nursing staff members."[17]

You have completed the section "Writing Standards for Perioperative Care."

SECTION 3

Writing Standards for the Emergency Department

Patients and their families who come to the Emergency Department are usually experiencing an unexpected severe illness or an accident resulting in health problems or needs requiring an immediate solution. Standards define the assessment, treatment, and care for patients' health problems in the Emergency Department. Another purpose for writing standards in the Emergency Department is to define the types of data needed by the police and the health department concerning problems affecting the safety of the patient and others in the community, as well as the data that must be documented regarding the assessment and treatment of the patient's health problem.

The characteristics (content and order) of the units of care must facilitate the treatment and care of the patient when speed is vital to the patient's outcomes. The essential characteristics of the units of care in the Emergency Department are:

1. The unit of care begins at triage and ends at discharge.

2. The standards must be written so that it is easy and efficient for the clinician to document what is required.

3. Documentation concerning equipment and supplies used in the diagnosis and treatment is required for third-party reimbursement agencies.

The patient and others involved in the emergency may be experiencing moderate levels of anxiety or are in crisis. A crisis can be defined as "a state that results when a person experiences a stress that is unmanageable and is threatening to his well being."[1] The person's traditional coping mechanisms are unable to deal with the situation, resulting in increasing anxiety.

The clinicians must implement the standards for the assessment and treatment of the patient's health problem(s) and assist in decreasing the stress of the persons in crisis until the treatment relieves the symptoms experienced by any person involved. Thus, all the units of care are implemented in a milieu of communication that:

1. Assists in minimizing the effects of or preventing crisis for the patient and his family and others that are involved by:
   a. Providing support
   b. Providing structure
   c. Reducing environmental stimuli
   d. Providing information
   e. Setting priorities
   f. Implementing interventions for stress-reduction

2. Encourages the patient to verbalize his perception of the emergency situation.

3. Assists the clinician to clarify aspects of the data needed to make a definitive medical and nursing diagnosis and provide appropriate treatment.

4. Enables the clinician to begin treatment while making further assessment.

Each unit of care will contain a chief complaint and a nursing diagnosis, plus the content and process standards for the following categories of standards. These categories of standards are the framework to be used for developing units of care in the Emergency Department.[2]

With the exception of "collection of evidence," all categories should be included in each unit of care. Collection of evidence has been listed as the last category because it is not used with all units of care. When it is needed, this category follows other assessments.

The categories are:

1. Assessment
2. Diagnosis, treatment, and care
3. Homegoing instructions
4. Patient's health status on discharge
5. Reimbursable items used in the diagnosis, treatment, and care
6. Emergency Department Log
7. Collection of evidence (as needed)

Examples of chief complaints, nursing diagnoses, and standards for each of the categories are as follows.

CHIEF COMPLAINT AND NURSING DIAGNOSIS

The assessment and examination of the patient begins with clarification of the chief complaint expressed by the patient and selection of a nursing diagnosis.

Chief Complaint	Nursing Diagnosis
Hallucinations	High Risk for Violence Self-Directed or Directed at Others[3]
Eye Injury/Inflammation	Potential for Visual Sensory-Perceptual Alteration
Headache	Pain Potential for Altered Thought Processes
Human/Animal/Insect bite	Potential for Impaired Tissue Integrity Potential for Infection
Back Pain	Pain Impaired Physical Mobility

Assessment

Assessments are essential throughout the patient's care and treatment:

    a. During triage
    b. Common to all units of care
    c. Related to a health problem

Examples of each type of assessment are as follows.

During Triage

Hemophiliac Crisis [4]

1. Assess:
   a. Bleeding (site)
   b. Bleeding: ( ) spontaneous ( ) traumatic
      (If traumatic, answer items c and d)
   c. Type of trauma
   d. Point of impact
   e. Previous bleeding episode
   f. Pre-hospital care: ( ) No ( ) Yes. If yes, type _____

2. Triage status: ( ) Non-urgent ( ) Urgent ( ) Emergent

Common to All Units of Care[5]

Level of Consciousness	*Mental State*	*Airway/Ventilation*
	( ) Alert	( ) Mouth to mouth
( ) Spontaneous	( ) Oriented	( ) Oropharyngeal
( ) Verbal	( ) Confused	( ) Bag mask
( ) Tactile	( ) Verbal stim.	( ) Valve
( ) Pain	( ) Painful stim.	( ) Esophageal airway
( ) Eye opening	( ) Unresponsive	
( ) None	( ) Appropriate for age	( ) Oxygen _____ LPM
		( ) Mask ( ) Cannula

Verbal Response	*Pupils* ( ) Equal		*Skin* ( ) Normal
( ) Oriented	R	L	( ) Pale (Turgor):
( ) Confused	( ) Reactive	( )	( ) Cyanotic ( ) Good
( ) Inappr. Words	( ) Nonreactive	( )	( ) Sweaty ( ) Poor
( ) Incomp. Words	( ) Fixed	( )	( ) Hot
( ) Appropriate for age	( ) Dilated	( )	( ) Cool
( ) None	( ) Constricted	( )	( ) Flushed
	( ) Cataract	( )	( ) Mottled

Respiratory Effort	*Chest*		*Abdomen*
( ) Normal	R Clear Pain	L	( ) Normal ( ) Tender
( ) Shallow	( ) Crackles	( )	( ) RUQ ( ) LUQ
( ) Retractive	( ) Rales	( )	( ) RLQ ( ) LLQ
( ) Rapid	( ) Wheezes	( )	( ) Epigastric Region
( ) None	( ) Decreased	( )	( ) Rigid
	( ) Rhonchi	( )	( ) Distended

Capillary Return	R	L	
	( ) Absent	( )	( ) Bowel Sounds _____
( ) Normal			Hyper _____ Hypo _____
( ) Delayed			Absent _____
( ) Cyanotic			Normal _____

Related to a Health Problem

Example: Eye injury and/or inflammation.[6]

1. Assess for:
   a. Diplopia
   b. Blurred vision
   c. Loss of part or all of a visual field
   d. Pruritis
   e. Burning
   f. Photophobia
2. Test visual acuity
3. Assess if present in one or both eyes:
   a. Redness
   b. Periorbital edema
   c. Periorbital ecchymosis
   d. Crepitus upon palpation of the orbital rim
   e. Purulent drainage
   f. Injury to everted eyelid
   g. Hyphema
   h. Subconjunctival hemorrhage
   i. Foreign object

    j. Laceration

    k. Chemical burn

Diagnosis, Treatment, and Care Related to:

    a. Burns

    b. Anaphylactic shock

    c. Fractures

Homegoing Instructions[7]

a. Discharge instructions issued?	( ) Yes ( ) No
b. Discharge instructions understood?	( ) Yes ( ) No

Examples of topics:

    a. Care of wound

    b. Medication administration

    c. Observations to report to the physician

Patient's Status on Discharge[8]

Example: Joint extremity injury/Fractures

a. Pulses to affected extremity palpable?	( ) Yes ( ) No
b. Capillary refill less than 35 seconds?	( ) Yes ( ) No
c. Color of extremity adequate?	( ) Yes ( ) No
d. Sensation to extremity adequate?	( ) Yes ( ) No
e. Able to use crutches?	( ) Yes ( ) No

Stable   *Non-stable*

( ) Home   Admit to _____

( ) Dr.'s office _____

( ) Nursing home

Method of transportation upon discharge:

( ) Ambulatory   ( ) Stretcher

( ) Wheelchair   ( ) Ambulance

Accompanied by whom (Relationship) _____

Reimbursable Items

    a. Debridement ointments/creams
    b. Wound care: cleansing solutions, anesthetics, and dressings
    c. Nasogastric tube
    d. Infusions and blood products

Emergency Department Log[9]

These data are necessary to ensure the patients are receiving the most efficient care possible:

    a. Time patient was triaged
    b. Time patient was seen in the treatment room
    c. Time seen by an Emergency Department physician
    d. Time the family physician was notified
    e. Time seen by the family physician
    f. Time police arrived
    g. Signature and badge number of the police officer, etc.
    h. Time discharged/admitted
    i. Caregiver's signature(s)
    j. Physician's signature

Collection of Evidence

    a. Child abuse
    b. Rape
    c. Battery

Two examples of units of care for the Emergency Department are:

    4. Sexual Assault/Rape[10]
    5. Psychiatric Disorders[11]

The category of standards for each group of standards will be labeled with its number and name throughout the example.

CHIEF COMPLAINT: SEXUAL ASSAULT/RAPE

Nursing Diagnosis: Potential for: (1) powerlessness (2) rape trauma syndrome (3) spiritual distress (4) infection.

Assessment: During Triage

Temp _____ P _____ R _____ B/P_____/_____
When and where assault took place:
Date: _____ Time: _____
Weapon involved? ( ) Yes ( ) No
Penetration: ( ) Oral ( ) Rectal ( ) Vaginal
Onset of Menarche: _____
LMP: _____gr _____ para _____ Ab
Contraception Method: __ Bathed since assault? ( ) Yes ( ) No Time:__
Last time voided _____ Bowel movement _____
Last time patient had sexual intercourse _____
Race of sexual partner _____
Patient seen by sexual assault nurse? ( ) Yes ( ) No
Name _____
HIV: ( ) Yes ( ) No
STD: ( ) Yes ( ) No
Triage Status: ( ) Non-urgent ( ) Urgent ( ) Emergent
Triage Nurse Signature: _____

Related to a Health Problem

1. Bruises	( ) Yes ( ) No
2. Lacerations	( ) Yes ( ) No
3. Contusion	( ) Yes ( ) No
4. Abrasions	( ) Yes ( ) No
5. Bite marks	( ) Yes ( ) No
6. Scratches	( ) Yes ( ) No
7. Vaginal discharge	( ) Yes ( ) No
8. Rectal tears/lac	( ) Yes ( ) No
9. Vaginal tears	( ) Yes ( ) No
10. Hematomas	( ) Yes ( ) No

Assessment Common to All Units of Care

- Vital signs
- Pattern documented after initial assessment until discharge

Assessment Related to a Health Problem

- Glasgow Coma Scale, Pupillary Reaction, Motor and Sensory Function
- Pattern documented after initial assessment until discharge

Diagnosis, Treatment, and Care Related to the Patient's Health Problem

For each of the interventions listed that are appropriate for this patient, list the time administered and the patient outcomes.

Lab	*Results:*
( ) CBC	_____
( ) SMA—24	_____
( ) VDRL	_____
( ) HIV (Need consent signed)	_____
( ) UCG	_____
( ) Serum HCG	_____
( ) UA	_____
( ) Vaginal Exam per: _____	Results: _____
( ) GC Culture	_____
( ) Chlamydia Culture	_____
( ) Gram Stain	_____
( ) Culture	_____
( ) Rectal: _____	Results: _____
( ) GC Culture	_____
( ) Chlamydia Culture	_____
( ) Gram Stain	_____
( ) Culture	_____
( ) Oral: _____	Results: _____
( ) GC Culture	_____
( ) Chlamydia Culture	_____

( ) Gram Stain _____

( ) Culture _____

Diagnosis, Treatment, and Care Related to the Patient's Health Problem

Medication Administration—for each medication include:
  a. Time administered
  b. Medication and dosage
  c. Route
  d. Site
  e. Administered by
  f. Effects

If a patient has been given a medication by intramuscular injection, there is a 30-minute wait to see the effect of the medication before discharge.

Diagnosis, Treatment, and Care Related to the Patient's Health Problem

IV Fluids/Blood Products Infused—for each infusion include:
  a. Time administered
  b. Solution
  c. Amount
  d. Site
  e. Total infused

Collection of Evidence

( ) Fingernail scrapings _____
( ) Saliva sample _____
( ) Hair samples _____
( ) Pubic _____
( ) Head _____
( ) Penile secretions _____
( ) Blood _____
( ) Semen _____
( ) Clothing collected _____
Issued to: _____

Homegoing Instructions

a. Discharge instructions issued? ( ) Yes ( ) No
b. Discharge instructions understood? ( ) Yes ( ) No
c. Patient understands need for follow-up and reevaluation post trauma? ( ) Yes ( ) No
d. Patient is able to express feelings about assault? ( ) Yes ( ) No
e. Patient understands need for psychological consultation? ( ) Yes ( ) No

Patient's Health Status on Discharge

( ) Stable   ( ) Nonstable

( ) Home   Admit to hospital room _____

( ) Dr.'s office _____   Transferred to: _____

( ) Nursing home

Method of transportation upon discharge:

( ) Ambulatory   ( ) Stretcher

( ) Wheelchair   ( ) Ambulance

Accompanied by whom (Relationship) _____

AMA?   ( ) Yes ( ) No

AMA Form Completed? ( ) Yes ( ) No

Reimbursable Items Used in the Diagnosis, Treatment, and Care of the Patient

• Collection of Evidence Kit

Emergency Department Log

These data are necessary to ensure the patients are receiving the most efficient care possible:

a. Time patient was triaged
b. Time patient was seen in the treatment room
c. Time seen by an Emergency Department physician
d. Time the family physician was notified
e. Time seen by the family physician
f. Time police arrived
g. Signature and badge number of the police officer, etc.

h. Time discharged/admitted
i. Caregiver's signature(s)
j. Physician's signature

CHIEF COMPLAINT:
PSYCHIATRIC DISORDERS

Nursing Diagnosis: Potential for: (1) anxiety (2) ineffective individual coping (3) fear (4) social isolation (5) disturbance in self-concept (6) sensory-perceptual alteration (7) spiritual distress (8) violence (9) impaired thought processes (10) alteration in nutrition (11) sleep pattern disturbance (12) impaired verbal communication (13) injury. (Select one or more nursing diagnoses.)

Assessment: During Triage

Temp _____ P _____ R _____ B/P _____/_____
History

Anxiety/Panic	( ) Yes ( ) No
Acute Psychosis	( ) Yes ( ) No
Paranoia	( ) Yes ( ) No
Aggressive Violent Behavior	( ) Yes ( ) No
Manic Depressive	( ) Yes ( ) No
Depression	( ) Yes ( ) No
Suicidal	( ) Yes ( ) No

(must have consult by a psychiatrist)

Bipolar Disorder	( ) Yes ( ) No
Previous hospitalizations	( ) Yes ( ) No

Where/When: _____

Substance Abuse

Alcohol ( ) Yes ( ) No

Drugs ( ) Yes ( ) No

When last used _____ Quantity _____
Comment: _____
Triage Status: ( ) Nonurgent ( ) Urgent ( ) Emergent
Triage nurse _____ Signature _____

Assessment Common to All Units of Care

Level of Consciousness

( ) Spontaneous
( ) Verbal
( ) Tactile
( ) Pain
( ) Eye opening
( ) None

Mental State

( ) Alert
( ) Oriented
( ) Confused
( ) Verbal stim.
( ) Painful stim.
( ) Unresponsive
( ) Appropriate for age

Airway Ventilation

( ) Mouth to mouth
( ) Oropharyngeal
( ) Bag mask
( ) Valve
( ) Esophageal airway

( ) Oxygen _____ LPM
( ) Mask ( ) Cannula

Verbal Response

( ) Oriented
( ) Confused
( ) Inappr. Words
( ) Incomp. Words
( ) Appropriate for age
( ) None

Pupils ( ) Equal

R   L
( ) Reactive   ( )
( ) Nonreactive ( )
( ) Fixed   ( )
( ) Dilated   ( )
( ) Constricted ( )
( ) Cataract   ( )

Skin ( ) Normal

( ) Pale Turgor___
( ) Cyanotic ( ) Good___
( ) Sweaty ( ) Poor___
( ) Hot
( ) Cool
( ) Flushed
( ) Mottled

Respiratory Effort

( ) Normal
( ) Shallow
( ) Retractive
( ) Rapid
( ) None

Chest

R Clear pain L
( ) Crackles ( )
( ) Rales   ( )
( ) Wheezes ( )
( ) Decreased ( )
( ) Rhonchi   ( )
( ) Absent   ( )

Abdomen

( ) Normal   ( ) Tender
( ) RUQ   ( ) LUQ
( ) RLQ   ( ) LLQ
( ) Epigastric Region
( ) Rigid
( ) Distended
( ) Bowel Sounds _____
Hyper _____ Hypo _____
Absent _____
Normal _____

Capillary return

( ) Normal
( ) Delayed
( ) Cyanotic

Assessment Related to a Health Problem

Mental Health Assessment

Affect   ( ) Appropriate ( ) Inappropriate ( ) Flat
             ( ) Constricted
             Comment: _____

Thought   ( ) Logical ( ) Illogical ( ) Circumstantial
processes   ( ) Tangential ( ) Loose Associations
             ( ) Flight of Ideas ( ) Delusional
             ( ) Ideas of Reference ( ) Paranoid Ideation
             ( ) Preoccupied ( ) Difficulty concentrating
             Comment _____

Perceptions ( ) Hallucinations: ( ) Visual ( ) Tactile
             ( ) Auditory ( ) Olfactory ( ) Command
             ( ) Gustatory
             Comment: _____

Speech   ( ) Rapid ( ) Pressured ( ) Slurred
             ( ) Slowed Responses ( ) Mute
             Comment: _____

Suicidal   Past and present history: Motive, plans
ideations   attempts _____
             Comment: _____

Homicidal   Past and present history: Motive, plans,
ideations   attempts
             Comment: _____

History of   ( ) Cruelty to animals ( ) Firesetting ( )
violence   ( ) Violent outbursts
             Comment: _____

Memory   ( ) Recent ( ) Remote
             Comment: _____

Assessment Common to All Units of Care

- Vital Signs
- Pattern documented after initial assessment until discharge

Assessment Related to a Health Problem

- Glasgow Coma Scale, Pupillary Reaction, Motor and Sensory Function
- Pattern documented after initial assessment until discharge

Diagnosis, Treatment, and Care Related to the Patient's Health Problem

For each of the interventions listed that are appropriate for this patient, list the time administered and the patient outcomes.

( ) Suicidal precautions _____

( ) Name of psychiatrist contacted _____

( ) Provide quiet room _____

( ) Restraints required: ( ) Yes ( ) No   Reason _____

( ) Patient medicated: ( ) Yes ( ) No

( ) Thorazine _____ mg
   Sedation achieved: ( ) Yes ( ) No

( ) Haldol _____ mg
   Sedation achieved: ( ) Yes ( ) No

( ) Cogentin _____mg
   Extrapyramidal symptoms relieved: ( ) Yes ( ) No

( ) Benadryl _____ mg
   Extrapyramidal symptoms relieved: ( ) Yes ( ) No

( ) Xanax _____ mg
   Anxiety decreased: ( ) Yes ( ) No

( ) Other medication _____ mg
   Result:

Narrative: _____

Diagnosis, Treatment, and Care Related to the Patient's Health Problem

Medication Administration— for each medication include:

1. Time administered
2. Medication and dosage
3. Route
4. Site
5. Administered by
6. Effects

If a patient has been given a medication by intramuscular injection, there is a 30-minute wait to see the effect of the medication before discharge.

IV Fluids/Blood Products Infused—for each infusion include:

1. Time administered
2. Solution
3. Amount
4. Site
5. Total infused

Homegoing Instructions

Discharge instructions issued? ( ) Yes   ( ) No
Discharge instructions understood? ( ) Yes ( ) No

Patient's Health Status on Discharge

Behavior controlled?   ( ) Yes ( ) No

Thought processes cleared?   ( ) Yes ( ) No

Medically stable?   ( ) Yes ( ) No

( ) Stable   ( ) Nonstable

( ) Home   Admit to hospital room _____

( ) Dr.'s office _____ Transferred to: _____

( ) Nursing home

Method of transportation upon discharge:

( ) Ambulatory   ( ) Stretcher

( ) Wheelchair   ( ) Ambulance

Accompanied by whom (relationship) _____

AMA?   ( ) Yes ( ) No

AMA form completed?   ( ) Yes ( ) No

Reimbursable Items Used in the Diagnosis, Treatment, and Care of the Patient

1. ( ) Number of syringes used
2. Wound dressing:
    a. ( ) Neosporin ointment
    b. ( ) Betadine ointment

c. ( ) 4 × 4

d. ( ) Kling bandage

Emergency Department Log

Time to room: _____Time ED physician notified: _____
Time seen by ED physician: _____
Time family physician notified: (first call) _____ (second call) _____
Time seen by family physician: _____
Time police arrived: _____ Signature: _____
Time discharged: _____

SUMMARY

When writing standards for the Emergency Department, the units of care begin with triage and end with the Emergency Department Log. Because of the speed required to assess the patient and begin treatment and care, the triage nurse selects the unit of care related to the patient's chief complaint or nursing diagnosis. As the clinicians are working with the patient, the legal documentation of what is done for the patient can be rapidly and accurately documented on the patient's plan of care throughout the patient's experience in the Emergency Department. You have completed the section "Writing Standards for the Emergency Department."

SECTION 4

Writing Standards for Discharge Planning

Discharge planning is an important component of care, regardless of the type of agency to which the patient is admitted. You want to prevent the following causes of delay in discharge of the patient:[1]

1. Assessment inadequate
2. Referral forms not sent and/or incomplete
3. Delay in lab tests/procedures and/or results not received by clinicians
4. Delay in consultations and/or results not received by physicians

5. Interdisciplinary planning not done and/or some members of the team absent
6. Inadequate communication among clinicians/departments
7. Patient's needs on discharge assessed too late or not assessed

There should be *three* aspects to discharge planning:

1. Initial assessment
2. Interdisciplinary planning
3. Preparation for discharge

INITIAL ASSESSMENT

The initial aspect of discharge planning occurs with the interdisciplinary assessment of the patient on admission to the facility. This initial contact with the patient should include assessment of the patient's health status to identify his potential needs on discharge, including the characteristics of the home environment and support services being used by the patient prior to admission.

Examples of these assessment items are:[2]

- Living arrangements:
  _____ Lives alone
  _____ Lives with family member(s); number _____ relationship _____
  age _____ any disabilities?_____
  Other—relationship _____
  age _____ any disabilities? _____
- Power of attorney _____ If yes, in whose name _____
  Phone number _____ Relationship _____
- Do any of the person(s) living with the patient have problems requiring the attention of a health professional? _____
- Type of dwelling
  Own home _____ one-story _____ two-story _____
  Family member's home _____ relationship _____
  one-story _____ two-story _____
  Boarding home _____ Nursing home _____
  Other _____
- Describe the patient's setting in relation to his needs for assistance from others. _____

- Who assisted the patient with his needs? Describe.
  Family members _____
  Friends _____
  Community services _____
  Other _____
- Needs assistance with:
  Cooking _____   Household maintenance _____
  Personal care _____   Shopping _____
- Does anyone living with the patient need assistance with:
  Cooking _____   Household maintenance _____
  Personal care _____   Shopping _____
- On discharge, will the patient need assistance with:
  Bathing _____   Toileting _____
  Grooming/Dressing _____   Ambulation _____
- When the patient is discharged, will he have transportation?
  Yes ____ No ____ If yes, Self ____ or Family member ____ Phone ____
  If no, type of transportation needed? _____
- Prior to admission did the patient require services from: (Describe)
  Visiting Nurse/Community Health _____
  Outpatient physical/psychiatric therapy _____
  Homemaker service _____
  Meals delivered _____
  Physical Therapy _____
  Occupational Therapy _____
  Respiratory Therapy _____
  (Include types of community resources available)
- Prior to admission did the patient need to:
  Follow a special diet _____
  Take medication(s) _____
  Use special devices for:
      Eating _____
      Personal care _____
      Ambulation _____
- Will there be someone in the patient's home setting who will be caring
  for the patient on discharge? ____ Name _____
  Relationship _____ Phone _____
  Age ____ Any disabilities? _____

INTERDISCIPLINARY PLANNING

If the initial assessment reveals the patient will require assistance after discharge, a unit of care, *Discharge Planning Alert*, is placed on the patient's plan of care.

This unit of care becomes a signal for clinicians to review the patient's initial assessment and to identify whether they need to be involved in the discharge planning for this patient. The clinicians can then complete their specific assessments related to discharge needs. (The clinicians who will be contributing interventions to the patient's plan of care must assess the patient so that they bring their discipline's expertise to the planning process.)

DISCHARGE PLANNING ALERT

This patient will need further assessment related to needs for care/assistance after discharge in the following:

- Living arrangements ( ) Yes ( ) No
- Power of attorney ( ) Yes ( ) No
- Type of dwelling ( ) Yes ( ) No
- Requires assistance from others ( ) Yes ( ) No   Type _____
- Assistance required by others in home ( ) Yes ( ) No   Type _____
- Need for transportation ( ) Yes ( ) No
- Community services needed before admission:
    - a. Homemaker   ( ) Yes ( ) No
    - b. Meals delivered   ( ) Yes ( ) No
    - c. Respiratory Therapy   ( ) Yes ( ) No
    - d. Physical Therapy   ( ) Yes ( ) No
    - e. Occupational Therapy   ( ) Yes ( ) No
        (Include types of community resources available)
- Needs special devices ( ) Yes ( ) No

An interdisciplinary conference including the patient and his family is held to identify the interventions that will be added to the patient's plan of care to ensure he will have the resources needed on discharge. The goals of the plan are to:

1. Link inpatient resources to the patient's needs
2. Identify the community resources needed by the patient

3. Assign responsibility for accessing these resources and dates for completion
4. Write referrals to the community agencies

Then, a unit of care, *Discharge Planning and Referral*, identifying the needs of the patient, the standards for accessing community resources, and the clinicians who are responsible for the discharge planning, is placed on the patient's plan of care. The following example of a patient having an arthroplasty of the hip is an illustration of the use of this unit of care with a patient's plan of care.

PATIENT'S PLAN OF CARE

Surgical Procedure: Arthroplasty of the Hip

Goals

1. The patient will not experience preventable complications.
2. The patient and his family will understand the care of the patient after discharge.
3. The patient will understand Total Hip Arthroplasty (THA) precautions for all functional tasks.
4. Patient will be independent in THA exercise program.
5. Patient will ambulate with _____/without _____ assistance.
6. Patient will be able _____/require assistance _____ to transfer.

Process Standards

Nursing Diagnoses: (1) Impaired Skin Integrity, (2) Impaired Physical Mobility, (3) Pain, (4) Potential for Injury, (5) Altered Pattern of Elimination, Altered Nutrition, Less Than Body Requirements (6) Knowledge Deficit (7) Fluid Volume Deficit:[3]

1. Position the patient to prevent dislocation of the hip:[4]
   a. Abduction of the legs
   b. Head of the bed 45 degrees or less
   c. Supine or unoperated side
   d. Small pillow in lower back when in the supine position
2. Check vital signs q4h. Report significant changes to the physician.

3. Auscultate all lobes of both lungs qid. Report significant changes to the physician.

4. Neurovascular checks q____h. Compare the operated with unoperated leg. Report significant changes to the physician.

5. Administer medication for pain PRN. Report increase in pain to the physician.

6. Observe incision for inflammation and infection daily (redness, exudate, edema, and heat). Report significant changes to the physician.

7. Assist the patient to ambulate maintaining weight-bearing restrictions.

8. Observe patient's toleration of all activities (before and after activity):

   a. Degree of fatigue

   b. Degree of weakness

   c. Presence of dyspnea

9. Indwelling catheter. Catheter care q8h.

10. Intake and output.

11. Encourage intake of fluids to 3000cc, unless contraindicated.

12. Observe patient's nutritional intake at each meal. If nutritional intake is inadequate, notify the physician.

13. Antiembolic stockings.

14. Teach the patient/significant others:[5]

   a. Activity restrictions

   b. Symptoms/problems to report to physician

   c. Medications

   d. Antiembolic stockings

   e. Post-urinary catheter observations

   f. Prevention of constipation

   g. Nutrition

Physical Therapy: The patient will receive treatment in the Physical Therapy Department twice a day to implement the following treatment plan:

15. Total Hip Arthroplasty (THA) precautions

   a. Instruct patient in THA precautions.

    b. Review daily until the patient can verbalize the precautions.

2. Transfer training
    a. Transfer patient from a supine to sitting position.
    b. Transfer patient from bed to chair.
    c. Transfer patient from sitting to standing.

3. Progress range of motion and exercise as patient tolerates it
    a. Range of motion exercises
    b. Isometric gluteal, quadricep, and hamstring setting and ankle pumps

4. Begin gait training using appropriate assistive device with surgeon-ordered amount of weight bearing

5. Instruct patient in car transfer and stairs, as needed.

Outcome Standards

Before discharge at all times:

1. The patient is not experiencing preventable complications.
    a. Wound or joint infection
    b. Dislocation of the hip
    c. Thrombophlebitis
    d. Altered perfusion in the peripheral tissues

After discharge:

2. The patient can verbalize his/her care:
    a. Activity restrictions
    b. Symptoms/problems to report to physician
    c. Medications
    d. Antiembolic stockings
    e. Post-urinary catheter observations
    f. Prevention of constipation
    g. Nutrition

3. The patient can verbalize Total Hip Arthroplasty (THA) precautions for all functional tasks.

4. The patient is able to ambulate with ____/without ____ assistance.

5. The patient is able to transfer ____/will require assistance ____ to transfer.

The Discharge Planning and Referral Unit of Care is added to the patient's plan of care.

DISCHARGE PLANNING AND REFERRAL

Goals

1. All community agencies needed to provide treatment and care to the patient after discharge will be contacted no later than _____ days before discharge.
2. All referrals to community agencies needed to provide treatment and care to the patient after discharge will be completed no later than the day before discharge.
3. The patient and/or his family will receive a copy of his post-discharge teaching plan.

Process Standards

1. Physician's orders   *(Physician)*

Note: A physician's order is needed for most community agency referrals.

2. Referrals to the following community agencies:

Health Discipline

  a. Home Care Agency: *(Nursing)*
    1. To evaluate patient's health status
    2. To change patient's dressings and observe the character of the wound
    3. To reinforce teaching (arthroplasty plan of care)
    Contact made _____ Date _____
    Referral sent _____ Date _____

  b. Physical Therapy   *(Physical Therapy)*
    1. To reinforce Total Hip Arthroplasty precautions
    2. To continue transfer training
    3. To progress range of motion and exercise as tolerated by the patient
    4. To provide gait training
    5. To order ambulatory equipment and raised toilet seat
    Contact made _____ Date _____
    Referral sent _____ Date _____

3. Finances for a walker   *(Social Work)*
   Contact made _____ Date _____
   Referral sent _____ Date _____

4. Transportation to work/therapy   *(Social Work)*
   ( ) Patient's home
   ( ) Extended-care facility
   ( ) Post-discharge therapy
   Contact made _____ Date _____
   Referral sent _____ Date _____

5. Arrange for a meal to be delivered daily   *(Social Work)*
   Contact made _____ Date _____
   Referral sent _____ Date _____

6. Arrange for a Hospital bed in the patient's home   *(Social Work)*
   Contact made _____ Date _____
   Referral sent _____ Date _____

7. All referrals completed. Date _____

Outcome Standards

The day before discharge:

1. All agencies contacted.
2. All referrals completed.
3. The patient has a copy of the post-discharge plan.

In addition, the plan should include the dates when lab tests, consultations, and therapy will be completed. Those departments responsible for consultations, lab tests, and therapy should participate in the planning process to ensure the dates for these items are accurate. Those clinicians responsible for implementing the plan should review the status of the implementation of interventions and the patient's responses to these interventions to ensure the plan is being implemented.

The clinician who is the leader of the group monitors the implementation of the entire plan. When changes are made to the plan, the leader notifies the appropriate clinicians to make the needed adjustments in their interventions.

The contacts to community agencies can be made early in the patient's stay if the initial assessment clearly indicates the patient will need these resources after discharge. For example, Social Work can begin obtaining necessary financial resources, counseling with the home care providers, arranging possible transportation for health appointments, arranging for nursing homes, etc., if the initial assessment and UOC on the patient's plan of care has indicated such needs.

COMMUNICATION WITH COMMUNITY AGENCIES

The third stage of discharge planning is preparing referrals and making contacts with agencies that will be providing services to the patient. For the agency to provide services and to obtain reimbursement, a physician's prescription and a written referral are often necessary. By preparing the patient for discharge as soon as possible after admission, the necessary paperwork and forms can be obtained on a more timely basis.

A plan of care detailing the patient's care needs should be sent with each referral. By the day before discharge, all interventions related to obtaining resources for the patient's care after discharge are completed. The clinician who is the leader of the planning group verifies that all preparations have been completed for the patient's discharge.

SUMMARY

Discharge planning is a vital component of the patient's care plan to ensure continuity of care as the patient returns home or to another health facility. When verbal contacts or referrals from clinicians caring for the patient provide the essential information needed to plan his care in the future, the patient will most likely have a plan of care that meets his needs and care that results in positive outcomes. You have completed the section "Writing Standards for Discharge Planning."

SECTION 5

Writing Standards for Home Care

Standards are needed to define the care of patients in their home to ensure they experience positive outcomes.

The major goals that standards address in home care are:

1. Assessments of the patient's health status and progress
2. Interventions implemented in the home

3. Assisting patients to become as self-sufficient as possible[1]
4. Providing homemaking services when needed
5. Assisting the patient and/or family to obtain other community services when needed

ASSESSMENTS

The assessment of the patient on the initial visit serves three purposes. The first is to obtain information needed to design the patient's plan of care. The second is to ascertain if the patient meets the eligibility criteria of the home care agency, accrediting agencies, and third-party payer agencies. The third is to identify whether others in the home have a need for health care.

Additional assessments are done at each visit by the clinician to determine the patient's progress toward the outcome standards and to continue to verify the patient's elgibility.

INTERVENTIONS

The interventions implemented in home care may be the same as those implemented in acute care, such as changing the dressing of the patient and making observations concerning wound healing. Or, interventions may be implemented to assist the patient and/or family in modifying their lifestyle or the patient's environment to help the patient with his health problems.

TEACHING

One of the most important functions of the clinician during a home visit is to teach the patient how to learn to cope with his health problem. The clinician can observe how the patient is coping in his home environment and assist the patient in either using more effective strategies or in improving the strategies he is using. Because teaching is an integral part of all the care that is implemented in the home, the content standards for teaching should be included in all the units of care implemented in the home.

HOMEMAKER SERVICES

The patient may be able to manage his own care but not be able to maintain the home. Thus, homemaker services may be the essential elements in the patient's plan of care to assist the patient to recover from or cope with a health problem. If these services are needed by the patient, they should be included in the unit of care.

OTHER COMMUNITY AGENCIES

During the assessment of the patient or the implementation of the patient's plan of care, the clinician identifies the patient's and/or family's needs for services provided by other community resources. The following information is needed concerning each agency:

1. Services for the patient and/or family
2. The telephone number and address
3. Eligibility requirements
4. Type of payment accepted

This information is written in the unit of care or referenced to an associated list readily accessible by the clinician.

One of the challenges in providing home care is to document what is "reasonable and necessary" skilled care to meet the requirements of accreditation and to "convince third-party payers of the fiscal legitimacy of submitted claims."[2] Standards designed for home care need to include these requirements and the requirements for documentation of the care of the patient. The standards do not need to specify the style of documentation, but they need to include *what* needs to be documented (unless accrediting agencies or third-party payers specify a style or form for documentation).

Examples of units of care for home care are:

1. Admission of the Patient to a Hospice
2. Medication Administration in Home Care
3. Home Care of the Patient after a Hip Replacement

HOSPICE ADMISSION[3]

Goals

1. Baseline assessment data concerning a potential patient will be obtained to determine eligibility for admission.
2. Necessary admission forms according to agency policies will be completed.
3. Patient will be oriented to hospice routines.

Policies

1. To the extent that the resources of the agency permit, all eligible patients shall be accepted for services regardless of age, race, creed, sex, national origin, or financial status.
2. Referrals are initiated by a physician, nurse, social worker, or other health care professionals. Patients, their relatives, friends, or community agencies may also initiate a hospice referral. When possible, the patient is an active participant in the referral process.
3. The evaluation visit is conducted on all patients by the RN within 72 hours of the receipt of the referral. All exceptions will be documented.
4. Patients referred who do not meet the eligibility criteria are reviewed at the Interdisciplinary Team Meeting, and a decision will be made regarding acceptance.
5. The referring physician will be notified by the clinical supervisor when the patient does not meet the eligibility criteria.

Process Standards

1. A registered nurse records the referral information and obtains a signed Plan of Care from the referring physician.
2. Referral information is communicated to the clinical supervisor or designee who then assigns the patient to the appropriate RN based on the special needs of the patient and their geographic location.
3. During the evaluation visit, the patient's eligibility is assessed based on the following criteria:
   a. Meets established criteria for home care eligibility
   b. Prognosis of the illness is in terms of weeks or months. A prognosis of one year or less is acceptable.

    c. Patient and/or family understands the philosophy of hospice and agrees to accept such services.

    d. Patient has an identified caretaker who is willing to take responsibility for and coordinate care in the home.

    e. A licensed physician provides written orders.

4. RN obtains and records physical, psychosocial, and environmental data on the assessment form.

5. RN assesses all equipment and supply needs for appropriateness for the patient's use in his environment and records information on the assessment form.

6. Based on the evaluation and initial assessment, RN initiates the plan of care.

7. Following the social worker's evaluation, the patient and his identified problems are reviewed at the Interdisciplinary Team Meeting. The plan of care is then established and approved.

8. On the next visit, the patient is provided with the Patient Handbook, which contains the following information:

    a. Hospice philosophy

    b. Services provided

    c. Payment information

    d. Hours of services

    e. On-call system

    f. Statement of patient's rights

    g. Patient responsibilities

    h. Problems of compliant reporting procedure

9. The contents are reviewed with the patient.

10. The patient or patient's representative's signature are obtained on:

    a. Insurance forms

    b. Release of Information

    c. Consent for Care

    d. Acknowledgement of receipt of patient handbook

11. During the visit identify the need for other services and initiate the appropriate referral.

12. Address the patient's questions and concerns.

Outcome Standards

1. Within two visits, the eligible patient verbalizes understanding of agency procedures.
2. Documentation is completed within five days of the initial visit.
3. Communication takes place between the appropriate team members as needed.

MEDICATION ADMINISTRATION—HOSPICE AND HOME CARE[4]

Goals

1. To provide patients with information on drug therapy
2. To ensure prescribed medications are taken correctly

Process Standards

1. Assess and document on the Medication Form all patient medications identified during the initial visit and on subsequent visits:
   a. Check patient prescription and/or container label against the medications on the plan of care.
   b. Clarify discrepancies or questions with the attending physician.
   c. Identify contraindicated medications and contact the physician.
2. Assess and document on the Assessment Form all food and drug allergies identified during the initial visit.
3. Observe all medication for evidence of stability.
4. Instruct all patients on the purpose, use, side effects, and proper storage of their medications and document such in the medical record. A written medication list, if indicated, can be provided for the patient to follow in the home using the Medication Schedule Form.
5. Provide information and instructions on whom to contact in the event of problems or emergencies related to drug therapy.
6. Instruct on the proper disposal of infectious and hazardous substances in the home according to agency policy.
7. Teach appropriate handling of clean, sterile items, including the following:
   a. Safeguards against microbial contamination
   b. Appropriate storage methods

    c. Storage durations for solutions and sterile products

    d. Documentation of instructions provided to patient and caregivers

8. Monitor and document ongoing drug therapy, including the following:

    a. Therapeutic duplication in the drug regimen

    b. Appropriateness of dose, frequency, and route of administration

    c. Lab work to monitor the toxicity, side effects, and effectiveness of the drug regimen

    d. Potential drug and food interactions

    e. Need for communication with physician regarding concerns

9. Direct all questions pertaining to medications to the attending physician.

10. Administer investigational drugs following the established protocol. All other drugs must be FDA-approved.

11. Revise the Medication Form and the patient medication schedule when medication changes are ordered.

12. Document verbal orders for changes in medications in the care plan and confirm immediately with a written change in the patient's plan of care.

13. Consult current pharmaceutical reference materials available at each agency office for medication information or call Drug Information Center at _____.

14. Administer all injectable drugs as ordered by the patient's physician.

15. If a medication is administered and the possibility of an anaphylactic reaction exists, the staff nurse should be prepared to administer adrenalin chloride 1:1000 according to established agency policy.

Outcome Standards

Within _____ visits:

1. The patient and/or family verbalizes an understanding of medications.

2. The patient and/or family demonstrates correct medication administration.

3. Patient verbalizes the symptoms of drug interactions that need to be reported to the physician.

At all times:

4. The patient has lab work to monitor the effects of selected drugs.
5. Potentially harmful drug interactions are prevented or detected early and managed.

PATIENT'S PLAN OF CARE

Home Care after Arthroplasty of the Hip

The patient is recovering from hip replacement surgery. He has had a stroke and managed well with hemiplegia until he had his surgery. The interdisciplinary health team in the hospital sent referrals to community agencies after the patient's physician wrote the following orders for this patient's health care (see Patient's Discharge Planning and Referral Unit of Care on page 284).

1. Home Care Agency: Ten visits
   a. Evaluation of the patient's health status
   b. Care of the wound
   c. Bladder training
   d. Reinforcement of teaching

2. Physical Therapy: Twenty visits
   a. Provide gait training.
   b. Progress range of motion and exercise as patient tolerates it.
   c. Increase functional status in relation to gait and transfers.
   d. Instruct patient in going up and down stairs.

Goals

1. The patient will regain physical mobility and functional status in relation to gait and transfers.
2. The patient will experience a return to presurgical bladder function.
3. The patient's wound will heal without complications.
4. The patient's nutrition will be optimal.
5. The patient will understand how to prevent constipation.
6. The patient will understand how to prevent thrombophlebitis.
7. The patient will understand strategies to enhance sleep.

Process Standards

Physical Therapy:

1. Reinforce Total Hip Arthroplasty precautions.
2. Continue transfer training.
3. Progress range of motion and exercise as patient tolerates it.
4. Provide gait training.
5. Report significant changes to the physician.
6. Report changes in the patient's function to the Home Care Agency.

Potential Nursing Diagnoses:

(1) Impaired Skin Integrity (2) Impaired Physical Mobility (3) Potential for Injury (4) Altered Patterns of Urinary Elimination (5) Altered Nutrition, Less than Body Requirements (6) Potential for Constipation (7) Knowledge Deficit (8) Sleep Pattern Disturbance

At each visit:

A. Evaluate and document the patient's health status:
    1. Ability to do Activities of Daily Living
    2. Ability to void
    3. Characteristics of the wound
    4. Bowel pattern
    5. Ability to sleep
    6. Nutritional status
B. Report significant changes to the physician.
C. Report significant changes in the patient's ability to do Activities of Daily Living to the physical therapist.
D. Reinforce teaching:
    1. Activity restrictions
    2. Symptoms/problems to report to the physican and physical therapist
    3. Medications
    4. Application of anti-embolic stockings
    5. Care of the wound and observations related to it
    6. Bladder training
    7. Prevention of constipation
    8. Nutrition
    9. Prevention of infection

10. Use of assistive devices

E. Document the patient and family's responses to teaching.

Outcome Standards

Within _____ visits:

1. The patient regained physical mobility and functional status in relation to gait and transfers that is optimal for him.
2. The patient experienced a return to presurgical bladder function.
3. The patient's wound healed without complications.
4. The patient's nutrition is optimal for him.
5. The patient's bowel pattern has returned to presurgical status.
6. The patient verbalizes how to prevent thrombophlebitis.
7. The patient is experiencing his presurgical sleep pattern.

SUMMARY

The standards for Home Care assist the patient to meet goals for his treatment and care when he needs to receive the care at home or in the community. In addition to the process and content standards, these units of care must include the documentation necessary to establish the eligibility for these services. You have completed the section "Writing Standards for Home Care."

SECTION 6
Standards to Complete Examples in the Book

In the main body of the text the standards used as examples to illustrate the concepts in the different sections did not have the related process or outcomes with them. This section was designed to add those standards needed to complete the examples of units of care written throughout the book.

UNIT OF CARE

Potential for Pneumonia

(Example on p. 20)

Outcome Standards

At all times:[1]

1. The patient's expectorated secretions are normal (clear, colorless, odorless, of small quantity; not viscid, tenacious, or watery).*
2. The patient's breath sounds are clear in all lobes of both lungs.*
3. The patient performs his activities without fatigue or dyspnea.*
4. The patient's temperature is normal.*
5. The patient's arterial blood gases are within normal limits.*

*Patients who have abnormal responses due to preexisting pathology use admission baseline for comparing with outcome data.

Potential for Urinary Tract Infection

(Example on p. 58)

Process Standards

1. Encourage fluids up to 3000cc unless contraindicated.
2. Monitor intake and output q8h. Report significant changes to the physician.
3. Observe for increased temperature, chills, flank pain, urgency, frequency, and burning on urination q4h. Report to physician and obtain a urine culture.
4. Notify physician if urine has unusual characteristics such as blood, excessive sediment, foul odor, or inflammation around the meatus. If any symptoms present, obtain a urine culture.
5. Monitor lab results and report abnormals to the physician.
6. Monitor vital signs q4h for 48 hours, then q8h.

Potential for Falls

(Example on p. 131)

Outcome Standards

During admission assessment:

1. Each patient who has the potential for falling has been identified.
2. Intervention(s) to prevent falling are listed on the plan of care of each patient who has the potential for falling.

The Adult Patient Experiencing
Chronic Inefficient Airway Clearance

(Example on p. 137)

Outcome Standards

Before discharge:

1. The patient can describe measures to avoid infection.
2. The patient can describe the early indicators of respiratory infection.
3. The patient can explain measures to be implemented if early signs of infection are present.
   a. Takes antibiotics as prescribed
   b. Seeks professional assistance when needed
4. The patient states how to take his medications.
5. The patient can describe the side effects of his medications and what to do if they occur.
6. The patient explains how and when to alter dosage of his medications.
7. The patient can demonstrate measures to clear airway.
8. The patient can identify inhalants that irritate the airways.
9. The patient can describe how to eliminate these agents in his environment.
10. The patient can explain daily activities in relation to the need for rest and activity.
11. The patient identifies situations that precipitate bronchospasm and collapse of the airways.
12. The patient verbalizes modifications he is making in his lifestyle to cope with his health problem.
13. The patient verbalizes knowledge of services of community, state, and federal agencies that might be assistive to him and the criteria for their use.

Within _____ weeks:

1. There is an absence of respiratory infections.
2. There is improvement in the effectiveness of the patient's breathing:
    a. Decreased dyspnea
    b. Decreased fatigue
3. The patient verbalizes that his family is supportive of his changes in lifestyle (if there have been changes).
4. The patient and/or family is using community, state, and federal resources when needed.
5. The verbalizations of the patient and his family, co-workers, and others indicate the patient's relationships with others are positive.

Note: If these outcomes are not positive, the patient and his family are making progress toward these outcomes.

Altered Sensory Perception
Related to Auditory Hallucinations

(Example on p. 143)

Outcome Standards

1. The patient can identify that the voices he hears are not heard by others.
2. The patient is able to function (work, etc.) without being preoccupied with hallucinations.
3. The patient realizes that taking medication has a direct connection with elimination or reduction of hallucinations.
4. The patient informs staff when the hallucinations are increasing or decreasing.
5. The patient is able to remain focused on the current conversation and not respond to the hallucination for at least _____ minutes per shift/day.
6. The patient completes a simple task such as _____ on a *daily/weekly/monthly* basis.
7. The patient is able to work with family/staff and/or significant other(s) to identify at least _____ stressor(s) that may increase the frequency of hallucinations.

You have completed the section "Standards to Complete Examples in the Book."

NOTES

Writing Standards for the Care of Children

1. Dianne Charsha, clinical specialist at Shore Memorial Hospital, Somers Point, N.J., 1993.
2. Ibid.
3. Ibid.
4. Ibid.
5. Ibid.
6. Ibid.
7. Ibid.

Writing Standards for Perioperative Nursing

1. Goldman, Maxine A. *Pocket Guide to the Operating Room.*, p. 16, Philadelphia: F.A. Davis, 1988.
2. *Excelcare System Standards Manual*, p. 25. Latrobe, Pa., 1993.
3. Association of Operating Room Nurses. *AORN Standards and Recommended Practices for Perioperative Nursing.* Denver, Colo., 1992.
4. Walsh, Judy. "Postop Effects of OR Positioning," *RN*, Vol. 56, No. 2, p.52, February 1993.
5. Goldman, op. cit., p.9.
6. Ibid., p.10.
7. Ibid., p.6.
8. Ibid., p.221.
9. Ibid., p.249.
10. Nurses at Lake County Hospitals, East and West. Painesville, Ohio, 1992.
11. Ibid.
12. Ibid.
13. Drescher, Nadine I. "An Integrated Care Plan," *AORN Journal, 54,* 6, pp.1265–1270, December 1991.
14. Lake County, op. cit.

15. Ibid.
16. Ibid.
17. Chana, Cheryl Hacker. "Documenting the Nursing Process," *AORN Journal, 55,* 5, p.1235, May 1992.

Writing Standards for the Emergency Department

1. Mowad, Linda, and Ruhle, Diane. *Handbook of Emergency Nursing: The Nursing Process Approach*, p.18. Norwalk, Conn: Appleton and Lange, 1988.
2. Cantu, Loretta, Alejandro, Mary, and the Emergency Department Nurses at McAllen Medical Center, McAllen Texas.
3. Carpenito, Lynda Juall. *Nursing Diagnosis.* New York: J. B. Lippincott Co., 1993.
4. Cantu, op. cit.
5. Ibid.
6. Ibid.
7. Ibid.
8. Ibid.
9. Ibid.
10. Ibid.
11. Ibid.

Writing Standards for Discharge Planning

1. Edwards, Julie, Reiley, Peggy, Morris, AnneMarie, and Doody, Joan. "An Analysis of the Quality and Effectiveness of the Discharge Planning Process," *Journal of Nursing Quality Assurance, 5,* 4, July 1991.
2. Ibid.
3. Carpenito, op. cit.
4. Thompson, June M., McFarland, Gertrude, K., Hirsch, Jane E., and Tucker, Susan M. *Mosby's Clinical Nursing* (3d ed.) p.412. St. Louis: C.V. Mosby Co.
5. Suddarth, Doris Smith. *The Lippincott Manual of Nursing Practice* (5th ed.), p.797. New York: J. B. Lippincott Co., 1991.
6. Mourad, Leona. *Orthopedic Disorders*, p.236. St Louis: Mosby Yearbook.

Writing Standards for Home Care

1. Williams, Rosie. "Nurse Case Management: Working with the Community," *Nursing Management 23,* 12, p.34, December 1992.
2. Sutton, Sunny. *Home Health Nursing Manual: Procedures and Documentation* (Preface). Baltimore: Williams and Wilkins, 1988.
3. Weaver, Robin, and the nurses in the Allegheny Home Care and Allegheny Hospice. *Medication Standard.* Pittsburgh, Pa., 1992.
4. Ibid. Allegheny Hospice Admission Standard.

Standards to Complete Examples in the Book

1. Wilson, Susan, and Thompson, June. *Respiratory Disorders*, p.184, St. Louis: Mosby Yearbook.

Index